THE
ENDURANCE
HANDBOOK

THE
ENDURANCE
HANDBOOK

How to Achieve Athletic Potential, Stay
Healthy, and Get the Most Out of Your Body

DR. PHILIP MAFFETONE

FOREWORD BY

TAWNEE PRAZAK, MS, CSCS

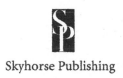

Skyhorse Publishing

Skyhorse Publishing books may be purchased in bulk at special discounts for sales promotion, corporate gifts, fund-raising, or educational purposes. Special editions can also be created to specifications. For details, contact the Special Sales Department, Skyhorse Publishing, 307 West 36th Street, 11th Floor, New York, NY 10018 or info@skyhorsepublishing.com.

Skyhorse® and Skyhorse Publishing® are registered trademarks of Skyhorse Publishing, Inc.®, a Delaware corporation.

Visit our website at www.skyhorsepublishing.com.

10 9 8 7 6 5

Library of Congress Cataloging-in-Publication Data is available on file.

Cover design by Qualcom Designs
Cover photos: Thinkstock

Print ISBN: 978-1-63220-498-1
Ebook ISBN: 978-1-63220-867-5

Printed in the United States of America

CONTENTS »

« CONTENTS »

FOREWORD »

I first found out about Dr. Phil Maffetone and the Maffetone Method through my podcast, Endurance Planet, in which my co-host—a coach and former professional triathlete himself—introduced me to Phil's aerobic-based heart-rate training. The concept, while nothing new in 2012, resonated with our podcast fans and more so it resonated with me. I read everything I could on the Maffetone Method to become an expert. Meanwhile, fans of our podcast began submitting dozens of questions asking everything you can imagine about the Maffetone Method, or "MAF" as it's commonly called for short (in fact, MAF stands for "Max Aerobic Function" and is not just Maffetone's name abbreviated). That year it's as if MAF had a rebirth on Endurance Planet, helping a whole new generation of endurance athletes understand how to reach new levels of performance and health (complete with the standard frustrations of athletes having to "run slow to get fast"). To this day, we address MAF so frequently on Endurance Planet that it's often accompanied with a laugh—"yup, another MAF question"—and it makes sense as to why: Everyone wants help on figuring out their unique path with the MAF approach because it's not a one-size-fits-all approach.

I eventually reached out to Phil asking him to be a guest on the podcast, and upon our first meeting and podcast recording—via Skype video—we quickly bonded and a friendship evolved. We continued podcasting together, and our chats would always run much longer than what was actually recorded for the show.

I am also an endurance coach and triathlete, and getting to know Phil and his work was greatly influential in molding my style of coaching as well as making me the athlete I wished to be. I was captivated by Phil's ability to listen, observe and assess people—myself included! (It's like he knows me better than me at times!) His wisdom and depth of knowledge are so vast, yet his presence is laid-back and casual. As a clinician who's so dedicated to collecting data and taking objective measurements, he's equally a free spirit and has a tendency to go "off the grid" to do his thing—something we should all mimic in effort to let go of being a chronically connected, go-go-go society. Phil's lifestyle is a testament that he's practicing what he preaches— he lives with low stress, he eats incredibly well even gathering food from his own garden, he moves and exercises in a way that keeps him strong and intact, and he has talents and hobbies that expand way beyond sport including his musical prowess.

While my coaching career does not span as many decades as Phil's does (but it will!), I am deeply ingrained in the endurance sports world, and it's clear to me we need more coaches and athletes to consider (and hopefully adopt) Phil's principles in their practices and lives. All too often I observe athletes—whether pro or amateur—wrecking their bodies in search of some extreme level of performance (usually, there's a coach somewhere supporting it), and at first it seems promising with some decent results, but eventually those athletes are unable to reach or hold on to those extremes because the body gives out in some form: injury, hormonal disruption, or some combination or manifestation that ultimately leads to a decrease in performance. This is an important concept you'll hear Phil discuss in this book.

To be perfectly honest, I've been there. As an athlete, I have made the mistake of doing more volume and intensity than what was healthy for my body. I eventually realized this, and even when I scaled back to MAF-based training I still found myself deeply evaluating my lifestyle and stress levels in order to fully recover and become healthy and stronger again.

And that's the thing about the Maffetone Method: It's all connected. It's all related. Athletic performance, health and lifestyle—they are all intertwined. With MAF, you can't hide behind poor health, and you can't hide behind bad habits. If you try, this method will wave its big fat red flags at you, namely the inability to improve at your MAF heart rate. In fact, the Number One reason people get frustrated and give up on MAF is that they're not able to go faster at the MAF heart rate. But it's not because MAF was wrong for them; it's because they didn't look deeper to solve underlying lifestyle problems that were causing this block.

Additionally, athletes and coaches will often argue that more intensity is needed than what's offered in the Maffetone Method. As such, many training programs and coaches dish it out under the notion that in order to perform better and/or to be the best *you must train harder, longer, take minimal recovery until you're back at it . . . and your health? Worry about that at some other time in life, they say, because sacrificing health now is OK; it's what it takes to get better.* Right? Wrong. Sadly, many athletes (and coaches) choose performance at the cost of health. We're constantly taught to adopt a mindset of "no pain, no gain" and go until you crash.

But it doesn't have to be this way to be successful.

If your body is in sync and in tune, then the Maffetone Method is a beautiful thing—just look at the success of six-time Ironman World Champion Mark Allen or my podcast co-host, Tim Luchinske, who was a talented professional triathlete-turned-ultrarunner, who's been top-10 in the Ironman World Championships, and in 2012 was overall winner of the grueling Leadman Ultra Series—no easy feat.

The Maffetone Method is the only training system I know of that promotes optimal performance *and* health, while remaining incredibly individual. When I coach athletes with the Maffetone Method it leads us to discovering more about that person as a whole, and we can collaborate to find their unique path to success. It forces you to evaluate your life, your health, your relationships, and so on, and sometimes the answers aren't clear—sometimes they're surface aspects of your existence that are tough to face and commit to changing, but you know you need just that. In that sense, it's not an easy training program to follow despite a simple formula of 180 minus your age, and that's the target heart rate at which to train. The Maffetone Method is not like a Jack Daniels or Joe Friel program for runners or triathletes, respectively, in which you can literally cut and paste the workouts into your schedule. Phil himself says plenty of times he's not here to simply give you a weekly schedule to follow.

The intrigue of "figuring out" MAF is probably why our Endurance Planet podcast saw such a robust response with thousands of questions and comments on the Maffetone Method. MAF can be complicated and usually includes some lifestyle adjustments, but when you stick with it and give it a chance, the results yielded with the Maffetone Method can often be much sweeter than a training program that leaves you trashed and unable to be a quality, healthy person. I've seen it happen! For as many how-to questions I get on MAF, I also receive thank-you emails nearly weekly from podcast fans that discovered MAF through our podcasts, and with it found success. Personally, I've also seen the success in the athletes I coach, and in me. To this day, my podcasts with Phil remain some of the most popular shows ever recorded on Endurance Planet, a podcast that's been in existence since 2006!

If you are ready to commit to being your best in sport and in life, then dive in and Phil will teach you how to do that.

—**Tawnee Prazak, MS, CSCS**
www.coachtawnee.com
www.enduranceplanet.com

PREFACE »

The *Endurance Handbook* serves as a supplement to my other recent books on endurance sports. This new volume is based on my newer articles, lectures and answers to questions from many endurance athletes, along with other new information. It also stands alone as a book that contains important items for every athlete. Contained within these pages are insights, commentary, more observations and diverse explanations about the philosophy and details of endurance sports. The goal is to help you become a more fit and healthy athlete.

The foundation of optimal endurance sports development includes the necessity to be healthy, thus avoiding the common patterns of injury, fatigue, poor performance, and plateau resulting from brain and body imbalance.

This book can be most useful when reading through all the Sections. If you still seek additional information or want to refresh yourself or further explore a particular topic, three other books—also meant to be read in their entirety but just as important are commonly used reference books—include the following:

- *The Big Book of Endurance Training and Racing.*
- *The Big Book of Health and Fitness.*
- *1:59 The Sub-Two-Hour Marathon Is Within Reach—Here's How It Will Go Down, and What It Can Teach All Runners About Training and Racing*

Continue to enjoy and endure!

—**Dr. Philip Maffetone**

INTRODUCTION: WHAT EXACTLY IS THE MAFFETONE METHOD? »

For many years, athletes, health professionals, coaches and trainers, and others have talked, written, debated and discussed the Maffetone Method. As often happens, some of these discussions lose accuracy or become distorted, so I want to introduce myself again, so to speak.

Throughout my career I have received questions asking why, after closely reading one of my books or articles, there was no workout schedule to follow. Or, people ask, where is the structured diet plan, you know, the kind with calorie charts that is a staple of most weight-loss books?

I can understand their frustration. We live in a quick-fix society. Everyone is looking for that single, magical diet or miracle workout plan that will change their lives overnight. But this is fiction, and one that all the health and fitness magazines love promising their readers.

But the only way to make long-lasting changes with one's health and fitness is to think in terms of the individual. Meaning you.

After close to forty years of working with individuals of all ages, levels of athleticism, and persons with the widest possible spectrum of illnesses and personal goals, I've yet to find the best diet for all to follow, or the ideal training program. That's because neither program exists, despite new books coming out each year that offer the long sought-after answer.

And that is why I created a unique approach, which became known as the Maffetone Method, starting in the late 1970s when I began my private practice. It basically says that we're all different and unique in every one of our needs.

My method is simple yet vast because that's the nature of humans; it's a holistic approach to help the individual figure out what makes him or her tick.

By taking this journey you also grasp the responsibility of your own destiny: the reward is that you can be healthier than you've ever been, fit enough to reach your athletic goals, and live a life whose quality is high.

But what exactly is the Maffetone Method? It has certainly stood the test of time.

Often times, the simplest things are the ones most difficult to explain. My method helps you take charge of your own health and fitness—and succeed. Every animal on earth intuitively knows how to be optimally healthy, but humans have gone astray; getting back your instincts is one of the benefits of this process.

Most diet fads or treatments for various ailments address the end-result signs or symptoms, leaving the cause of the problem ignored. While this is the hallmark of our healthcare system and society—drug and health stores alike are full of products that offer people a way to treat their symptoms—it obviously doesn't usually correct the cause of the problem.

The Maffetone Method's approach encourages you to find the reasons for poor health and fitness, answering the many popular questions: How can you get faster? Why can't you lose weight? What is the cause of your pain? What's needed to reach your athletic potential? I can't tell you the answers to these vital questions, but I can help you figure it out. Virtually everyone is capable of succeeding, but it requires a different way of thinking, and giving up the endless search for that magic pill, the perfect diet or other one-size-fits-all ideas.

Even without a clear and concrete definition, I could easily describe how my so-called "method" evolved and was fine-tuned so that anyone could apply it. And that's what it is, an evolution of ideas for all to use. Knowing that individual assessment and treatment was a key to developing a successful practice, along with helping patients understand the importance of self-health care, it became obvious that certain patterns existed in those individuals who were not perfectly balanced (essentially everyone, including myself). These were physical, biochemical, and mental-emotional imbalances—complete with various signs and symptoms. These patterns provided vital information, which helped lead to quicker and more accurate evaluations, and faster therapeutic outcomes.

This process lead to asking specific questions about how the body was responding to, say, pain. In particular how and when it started, what makes it better or worse, how long it lasts, and other information that makes it easier to find the cause of the pain, and eliminate it.

These questions are a vital part of my style, and important tools anyone can use to find and fix physical ailments, metabolic imbalances, and other problems. It's important to know that pain, injury, ill health, and a plateau or worsening of athletic performance is abnormal—it means something has gone wrong. Your job is to find the problem and eliminate it, using many of the tools written about here and in *The Big Book of Endurance Training and Racing*.

In addition to questions about body function, self-tests are very important. By evaluating the body's response to adding or avoiding certain foods or specific workouts, for example, one can obtain valuable information to begin piecing together the details of an individualized program. This also helps develop the instincts and intuition we all already posses.

There are many different facets of health and fitness that also must work together to create optimum human potential—like you felt when you were younger and full of vigor. This approach is a way for an individual to more objectively look at his or her whole life, and address any and all factors that are not working most advantageously for optimal health and fitness. These factors include one's diet or nutritional status, exercise routine, and how physical, chemical, and mental stresses are best regulated.

In short, the Maffetone Method is not a cookbook plan, but an approach for athletes who want to think out of the box, be creative, individualize their approach to sports to maximize results, and to develop their natural talents for years to come. In other words, we must rely on our brains, which control the body's performance. In order to achieve this, a healthy brain is necessary.

Let's look at some other specific topics that make this unique system so distinctive.

Primum non nocere

This popular Latin phrase is translated, *First do no harm.* Virtually all those in healthcare know the edict, first leaning it as students. It is an imperative ethical principle taught worldwide that, unfortunately, may not always be followed in our modern day healthcare environment. It is one I have embraced throughout my career, and also an important component of my advice to athletes everywhere.

For athletes, this ideal can be summed up as follows: Whatever is done to promote fitness—training, competition, diet, equipment, etc.—must not impair ones health. Unfortunately, studies continue to show fit but unhealthy athletes in all sport, and in men and women in every age group, including professionals. Children are not spared. The problem has become an epidemic.

A side effect of this problem is that, while too many athletes push their bodies to achieve more fitness in hopes of better competitive performance, this may actually not occur, or in some cases occurs only short term, but often at the expense of years of poor health.

There is an apparent paradox seen in athletes who are fit enough to perform what appears to be great feats, but at the same time have low levels of health, rendering them vulnerable to injury, illness, disease, and sometimes death.

The story of the ancient Greek runner Pheidippides inspired the modern day marathon. He is known for dying after a long run to declare a battle's victory. Some of my boyhood memories are of athletes dying. It was difficult to grasp how heroes could suddenly drop dead. Ultimately, the study of human physiology brought the answer: they were remarkable fit, but unhealthy. Despite advances in healthcare, this unfortunate problem continues today as more endurance athletes train harder and longer. A later section of this book will address this topic in more detail. For now, it's important to emphasize that it is the number one feature of the Maffetone Method.

Self-Evaluation

Perhaps the most important regular routine for endurance athletes is testing one's level of sub-max performance.

For most endurance events, competition is accomplished at relatively low levels of intensity, especially when compared to a track and field competitor or even during a 5K race. Longer events are accomplished successfully at sub-max state. A marathoner, for example, may win while racing around 83 percent of his or her VO_{2max}; for an Ironman and other ultra events that number is closer to 70 percent of VO_{2max}. The faster one can train at a sub-max pace, the better the performance. So monitoring the progress of sub-max performance is imperative for ongoing success—if you're not improving at the aerobic level, competitive success will not be realized.

This means you should be running, biking, or otherwise going faster in your event at the same sub-max heart rate throughout the year. By evaluating yourself every month or so, using a heart rate monitor to measure performance, you take the guesswork out of your training.

If progress is not forthcoming, something in your lifestyle is blocking it. This could be poor fat burning reducing energy, physical imbalance affecting gait, chronic inflammation impairing metabolism, excess stress, or other factors that reduce ones physical economy. Some of these are reviewed below, discussed throughout this book, and *The Big Book of Endurance Training and Racing.*

Burning Body Fat

One specific goal of the Maffetone Method is to increase the burning of body fat to provide high levels of physical and mental energy, and prevent the accumulation of excess stored fat and weight. Most of the body's energy for daily living comes from the conversion of both sugar (glucose) and fat to energy (in the form of ATP). Some people rely on larger amounts of fat, with the result of high physical and mental vigor, improved health, and better all-around performance. Those less able to burn sufficient fat must rely more on sugar, resulting in less fat burning each day—a problem associated with reduced health, including low energy, increased body fat and weight, less endurance for daily living, and lower physical fitness.

An important reason for burning more body fat has to do with the fact that it fuels our endurance—specifically, the aerobic system of the body.

Balanced Physical Activity

The most important way to instruct the body's natural fat-burning capabilities is to train the aerobic system. By stimulating the full spectrum of slow-twitch muscle fibers, which rely on fat for fuel, improvements in the heart and lungs, increased circulation, and better brain function, also occurs. This also helps the joints, bones, ligaments, tendons, and muscles prevent injuries, avoiding chronic pain conditions in areas like the low back, knee, shoulder, wrist, and neck.

Without specifically training the fat-burning system, one could actually become aerobically deficient, a common syndrome associated with fatigue, increased weight and body fat, reduced immune function (since the aerobic muscle fibers are key site of antioxidant activity), physical injury, and hormonal imbalance.

Controlling Chronic Inflammation

Another important aspect of my method is addressing a key chemical condition that leads to serious illness. Most diseases begin in a seemingly benign way, without symptoms or signs, as chronic inflammation. The chemical imbalances that trigger this problem are easy to control with diet and lifestyle. Specifically, by balancing one's dietary fat intake by eating only natural fats and consuming certain foods—based on a person's individual needs—avoiding chronic inflammation is easy to accomplish. In doing so, many of the physical and mental problems seen in aging can be avoided, including cancer, heart disease, arthritis, diabetes, weak bones and muscles, and Alzheimer's.

Secrets to Stress Management

Learning how to avoid the ravages of physical, chemical, and mental stress is an important part of my approach. Finding the ideal diet, maintaining optimal nutrition, regular aerobic workouts, and other lifestyle factors that would normally lead to optimal health and fitness won't work if excess stress interferes. Since the human body and brain has a unique system that manages stress perfectly well, learning how to enlist these natural activities are vital—they include the brain's hypothalamus and pituitary, and the body's adrenal glands.

Sugar Addiction

One of the most common causes of chemical stress, leading to reductions in aerobic function and fat burning, and chronic inflammation is the consumption of sugar and other refined carbohydrates. These junk foods have become a staple in the diets of millions of people—but addiction prevents their elimination. More than any other food they directly interfere with one's ability to be healthy and fit, and develop endurance potential. In fact, one meal or snack of sugar or refined carbohydrate not only can turn off fat burning and significantly disturb hormones, but also switch on genes that cause disease.

These are some of the important topics that make up much of the Maffetone Method.

How can this method offer a personalized, truly individual approach for all people? By doing what I've done throughout my career—begin by assessment. Through self-evaluation with the help of questionnaires and self-testing, and learning about the inner workings of the body, individuals are guided through the simple process of determining their particular needs in all key areas of health and fitness, from diet and nutrition, to exercise and the regulation of stress. The end result is improved human performance—including better brain function, increased endurance, avoidance of illness and disease, unlimited energy, and for athletes, continuous competitive improvements without injury.

All this begins with you deciding a change is needed. You must take the first step in your long and wonderful journey. Throughout the years, I have seen and heard many wonderful stories of success using my methods. I'd be happy to hear yours.

THE SECRET OF ENDURANCE: AEROBIC SPEED

One of the basic foundations of endurance sports performance is the aerobic system.

It plays a key role in running, cycling, triathlon, cross-country skiing, rowing, and even team sports such as soccer, basketball, hockey, and many others. In fact, any event that lasts more than a minute, even if not continuous, has a significant component of endurance, with a marathon relying on the aerobic system for 99 percent of the necessary race energy.

In addition to long-term stamina for optimal performance, the aerobic system provides us with an important bonus: it builds our health. Aerobic muscle fibers support the physical body, helping to maintain muscle balance for stability, and create an optimal gait for better movement economy. In short, the aerobic system can literally correct and prevent mechanical injuries like a therapist. This allows our joints, bones, ligaments, tendons, fascia, and other soft tissues to function most effectively. And there's more.

In addition, aerobic muscle fibers contain our antioxidant system, helping our immune system protect the whole body from illness, wear and tear, and literally hold back the rapid rate of aging so often seen in athletes.

The massive network of blood vessels contained in the aerobic muscle fibers helps improve the cardiovascular system. By bringing more blood in and out of our organs, glands, and everywhere else, a better functioning body is the result.

By burning fat as its main source of energy, the aerobic system prevents the accumulation of excess stored body fat. This is more than an unsightly state for the body. In addition to risking chronic inflammation, an overfat condition worsens movement economy, so it costs more energy to run, bike, ski, swim, and perform other endurance activities. Just reducing stored body fat can significantly improve performance.

The aerobic system also helps take care of our anaerobic muscle fibers, so that when we need a burst of power and sprint speed, these muscle fibers are readily available.

The aerobic system allows us to move for many miles without fatigue. But don't be fooled by the term *slow-twitch*. When well developed, the aerobic system can move the body very fast: consider that many athletes can run at sub-six minute per mile pace or race a fast bike leg of an Ironman event while remaining aerobic.

In order to maximize aerobic potential—perform faster during sub-max training and racing—one must be familiar with the definitions associated with the aerobic system.

Aerobic

The term aerobic is so popular that most people think they know what it means, or so they say. When asked, many associate it with breathing, air, or oxygen. Or they confuse it with "cardio" at the gym, where you can also find aerobic dance classes and pool aerobics. In fact, the term *aerobics* is as relatively recent as related exercise. It's not even fifty years old, although humans have been doing it for millions of years. In the late Sixties, Dr. Kenneth H. Cooper, an exercise physiologist for the San Antonio Air Force Hospital in Texas, coined the term "aerobics" to describe the system of exercise that he devised to help prevent coronary-artery disease. Dr. Cooper originally formulated aerobic exercises specifically for astronauts, but soon realized that the same set of exercises—jogging, running, walking, and biking—are useful for the general public as well, especially those suffering from being overweight, which are more likely to develop various heart and other diseases.

Anaerobic

Like the balance of yin and yang, the aerobic system has a counterpart called anaerobic.

The anaerobic system is important for power and sprint speed. It relies on sugar (glucose) for energy, which is very limited. This glucose energy comes from three main sources: blood sugar (from the diet), glycogen (the stored form of glucose), and blood lactate (which is continually produced by our metabolism, even during aerobic training and at rest).

Sugar is converted to energy in the anaerobic muscles, sometimes called fast-twitch or white-muscle fibers. They are used for short-term power (such as weight lifting) and sprint speed (such as an all out 100 meter race). These attributes are used very little in endurance sports as anaerobic energy is very limited—relying only on this system won't even allow a one mile race to be completed.

We don't normally use *only* the aerobic or anaerobic systems—or only fat or sugar—during training and competition. For example, the anaerobic system is limited to about three minutes of energy and, to maintain fat burning for aerobic activity, sugar burning is also necessary. It's the mixture of these two fuels that supply us with optimal performance energy. When an endurance athlete fatigues in a race, it may be associated with the loss of available glucose necessary to sustain the conversion of fat to energy in the aerobic muscle fiber, or due to the inability to burn enough fat because of poor aerobic training.

Once you see the difference between aerobic and anaerobic, this knowledge can help build better health and fitness. In addition, training through the transition from an aerobic to anaerobic state is one to be avoided for much of an endurance athlete's yearly schedule. Yet the focus of many training programs is on reaching the lactate and/or anaerobic threshold. While these states may have value, trying to develop them before one obtains a great aerobic system can impair performance.

So which system—aerobic or anaerobic—is working in you right now as you're reading these words? The surprising answer is both. It's easy to see that aerobic activity is important all the time—to maintain various functions such as posture and movement, long-term, consistent energy, and circulation. But even though we're not sprinting or lifting heavy objects, the anaerobic system is always performing some basic tasks such as burning sugar. In fact, within the complex metabolic pathways of energy production, burning some sugar helps maintain fat burning. In addition, the anaerobic system is always prepared to take action if necessary—humans have a "fight or flight" mechanism waiting to act should the need arise.

The real question is which system is predominating—which are you relying on? Is your body burning mostly sugar and less fat? If this is so, your anaerobic system is the one turned on more than your aerobic body. While you may not notice this—particularly if it's an ongoing problem—but if your energy and endurance are not what they should be, you are vulnerable to aches and pains, body fat content is too high, or you're under too much stress, as the anaerobic system is connected with our fight or flight stress mechanism. In short, your health is compromised.

Instead, you want long-term energy to be free of fatigue, maximum support for your joints and bones, injury-free muscles, good circulation, and increased fat burning to slim down. You want both optimal health and great fitness.

Aerobic vs. Anaerobic Training

Certain training will provide benefits that will build the aerobic system long term. I refer to these simply as aerobic workouts, meaning they will provide the stimulus to improve fat burning for more energy, continuous physical support, improved blood flow throughout the brain and body, and reductions in body fat. Relatively easy activities, such as running, biking, swimming, and others can accomplish this if the intensity of these workouts is not too high. Your heart rate is an accurate indicator—lower heart rate exercise is aerobic while performing the same workout with a higher heart rate would be anaerobic.

This is where the issues get more complicated:

- In the short term, almost *any* activity can help build the aerobic system, even very hard efforts. But continue these kinds of training routines for too long and your body will break down from injury, fatigue, and ill health. You'll become a casualty of the fit but unhealthy crowd. Essentially, you become over-trained. (Even traditional weight-lifting program can produce some aerobic benefits *short term*.)
- In order to effectively develop the aerobic system to produce faster training and racing paces, diet plays a key role. Without a continuous supply of fat for fuel, aerobic function will be limited. The primary enemy of endurance is refined carbohydrates—sugar and flour. These ingredients make up too much of the diet of the average athlete. These foods must be eliminated if you want to be a great endurance athlete.

For a workout to be truly aerobic, you should be able to train the same way for many weeks and months with *continued, measureable benefits*. And, when you're finished each workout, you should feel great—not tired and never sore, and certainly not ready to collapse on your couch. Nor should you have cravings for sugar or other carbohydrates—your workout should program your body to burn more fat, not sugar. Burning too much sugar during a workout means it's anaerobic, using up stored sugar (glycogen). It can even lower blood sugar. The result is that you crave sweets.

In a laboratory or clinical setting, the process of fat burning can easily be measured with a gas analyzer—a device that measures the amount of oxygen you consume from the air, and the carbon dioxide your body expires (called respiratory quotient). With this information, one can determine quite accurately the amount of fat and sugar burned for energy at various heart rates.

As aerobic training progresses, fat burning increases at various heart rates from rest to higher levels. This reflects improvements in the aerobic system as indicated by the ability to run, bike, swim, or otherwise go faster at the same sub-max heart rate.

Aerobic Speed

As all aspects of the aerobic system develop, your endurance will improve. This means you will be able to move faster at the same sub-max heart rate—running, cycling, swimming, and performing any endurance activity faster and more efficiently at the same level of intensity. This amazing phenomenon will carry over to competition—you'll be able to go faster during anaerobic efforts too. (Obtaining your sub-max training heart rate, which I refer to as the MAF heart rate, is discussed later in this section.)

Initially, when first training the aerobic system, most athletes have to slow down, with only some having to train faster. Some speed up quickly, while others progress more gradual. Still others don't appear to make progress and remain stuck at the same slow aerobic speeds.

In those who progress too slow or make no improvements, it means something is wrong. It's natural for humans to get faster— we've been doing so for millions of years. Even within our own lifetime, development of the aerobic system should continue well into our thirties and even past age forty—unless something—some factor in your lifestyle—blocks the process.

The most common reasons for lack of aerobic improvement include intake of refined carbohydrates, choosing an improper training heart rate, excess physical, chemical, or mental stress, and combinations of these and other factors discussed here, and in my other books and articles. By removing these roadblocks, aerobic function will be unleashed as indicated by training faster at the same sub-max heart rate.

In addition to removing the factors that impair natural endurance development, there are two essential techniques that can help the body increase aerobic speed. The first is important for those just starting to build the aerobic system, and the second is for those who are already developing aerobic speed. These are referred to as *downhill aerobic workouts*, and *aerobic intervals*, reviewed below:

Aerobic Essentials

These two tools that help build the aerobic system are important for those first developing a base and who may be frustrated at the slower speeds. Likewise for those who have built a great aerobic base and are having a hard time keeping up with it—running, cycling, or other activities are difficult to continue because of the faster aerobic speed.

Downhill Aerobic Workouts

While building your aerobic base, you can speed the process by doing *downhill workouts*. I refer to these as such because I first employed them with athletes running downhill, but this workout can be used for many activities such as running, biking, and cross-country skiing. This workout allows you to go at a faster pace without the heart rate rising. It will allow you to train faster without becoming anaerobic, and also to develop more leg speed during base building.

For example, at a heart rate of 145, if you can run at a 9:45 pace on flat ground, then running down a hill at the same heart rate will force you to run much faster, perhaps at a 8:45 pace depending on the hill's slope and distance. A cyclist may be cruising at 15 mph, and on a nice long, but moderate, downhill might average 26 mph at the same heart rate.

Using a long downhill that's not too steep, you can train your brain to turn the legs over much more quickly than would ordinarily occur during a run on a flat course—all while staying aerobic. If you have a long steady downhill that takes you ten minutes or longer to complete, you can derive great neuromuscular benefits. It's important to be sure the downhill is not too steep a grade, which may force a runner to over-stride, putting too much mechanical stress on the feet, knees, hips, and spine. Even on the right grade, your stride length should be about the same as if you were on level ground. (It's also important to wear shoes that are a perfect fit.)

If the downhill run is short, such as five minutes, you can do *downhill repeats*, walking or slowly running up the hill while staying aerobic to start your downhill interval again. Some treadmills can be adjusted to slant downhill, which is a nice alternative for runners.

I often suggest one or two downhill workouts per week, on non-consecutive days, during the base period. Even though you're aerobic, this workout does add more good stress to your body, and it's best to assure recovery by not using the technique on consecutive days. When properly done, most athletes don't feel much different than they would after any other workout, but some may feel a slight or mild soreness in some muscles, indicating the new activity. *If it's painful or muscle soreness is significant the next day, something is wrong—poor mechanics, bad shoes, too steep a hill, or some combination of problems.*

This workout need not be very long—runners can go forty-five minutes while cyclists up to an hour and a half, including warm-up and cool-down. These workouts can help you further develop more aerobic speed.

Aerobic Intervals

Once you have achieved a higher level of aerobic speed by building a more effective aerobic system, it may become difficult or impossible for you to reach your aerobic maximum heart rate, depending on the type of workout and the course. This is due to an improved aerobic system enabling you to perform faster at the same heart rate—the increased fat burning provides you with more energy for running, biking, and so forth. This is most true in swimming, cycling, skating, or cross-country skiing. Some runners will also feel the difficulty in maintaining a six or seven minute per mile pace every day. At this stage of your development, you may be ready to add what I call *aerobic intervals* to your program.

Aerobic intervals enable you to train at your maximum aerobic heart rate for short periods despite the difficulty in maintaining that level of activity. You'll know when you're ready for aerobic intervals; riding, for example, at your maximum aerobic heart rate will be physically challenging—your heart rate won't exceed the maximum aerobic level but you'll physically have a difficult time maintaining it, or even reaching it because you'll have to ride or run faster than your comfort level. This is exactly the opposite of what you felt when first starting out building an aerobic base, and thought that the pace was too slow.

Since you won't easily be able to maintain your maximum aerobic heart rate for the whole workout, or if it's just too challenging for an everyday activity, you can perform a short interval at or near your maximum aerobic heart rate, slow down for a period of time, and then go back to the maximum aerobic level. This is much like traditional interval workouts, except it's all aerobic.

For example, if your maximum aerobic heart rate is 152, and you want to do an aerobic interval session on the bike for ninety minutes, here's a sample workout:

- A twenty-minute warm-up
- Ten-minute segments consisting of five minutes at a heart rate of 152 and five minutes at 120, repeated five times for a total of fifty minutes
- A twenty-minute cool down

Developing a great aerobic system that allows the body to perform faster feats with the same effort (i.e., the same sub-max heart rate)—which translates to faster racing—is best accomplished during a period of strict aerobic workouts. This "base" period of training is the foundation of building optimal aerobic speed and better endurance.

The Aerobic Base

In the Introduction I emphasized a primary factor in my approach: *First do no harm*. Were I to list a second place item to emphasize it would be this: *Build the best aerobic base*.

The training period during which an endurance athlete focuses strictly on developing the aerobic system over a period of three to six months, sometimes longer, is called the aerobic base.

One reason for a creating a great aerobic base is that many of those who accomplish it perform their best in competition immediately afterward. They also have better endurance longevity and few, if any, injuries, and are healthier overall without problems such as allergies, asthma, digestive dysfunction, and others. Moreover, a great base results in slimming down. This reduction in body fat levels often results in weight loss, too.

I first learned about the concepts of base building in the late 1970s by reading about famed New Zealand coach, Arthur Lydiard, who died in 2004. You can read more about my work with Arthur in *The Big Book of Endurance Training and Racing*.

Developing an aerobic base means building the body while *only* training at a sub-max training heart rate. The reason I emphasize exclusive aerobic training during this base period is because anaerobic training may interfere with the process.

It's now quite clear that anaerobic training can impair aerobic function. Those who don't recognize this factor may not define aerobic and anaerobic the same way as I do. A common question remains: Just how does anaerobic training, competition, or other physical, chemical, and mental stresses (which mimic anaerobic activity) interfere with aerobic development? There may be several mechanisms associated with this problem:

• Any type of excess stress can interfere with the aerobic system by raising the hormone cortisol. This stress response, often not obvious in many cases, can interfere with many physiological processes in the brain, muscles, and metabolism that are necessary to develop aerobic function and endurance.

• High cortisol levels, a common marker of overtraining, also increases insulin levels (just like dietary sugar and other refined carbohydrates do), inhibiting the fat-burning process necessary for aerobic muscles to work well.

• Anaerobic training can decrease the number of aerobic muscle fibers, sometimes significantly. This can happen in just a few short weeks.

• Anaerobic training can raise your respiratory quotient, meaning that fat burning is reduced and sugar burning is increased, encouraging further use of anaerobic function and less aerobic activity.

• Elevations in blood lactate, produced in much higher amounts during anaerobic training, may impair aerobic muscle enzymes, reducing aerobic function.

• Anaerobic training typically causes hunger and craving to consume more refined carbohydrates. This can increase insulin levels and further interfere with fat burning, reducing aerobic function.

The Aerobic Deficiency Syndrome

In many endurance athletes, the lack of sufficient aerobic conditioning can cause many signs and symptoms, including serious physical, chemical, and mental injuries. This problem is not unlike a nutritional deficiency such as low iron causing anemia.

This aerobic deficiency or ADS, already an epidemic in the general population because so many people are sedentary, exists in millions of endurance athletes. The reasons may be due to lack of aerobic base, excess anaerobic work (such as intervals, racing, traditional forms of weight lifting), nutritional and dietary imbalance, and others.

Here are some of the important signs and symptoms associated with ADS:

- **Fatigue.** This is a very common complaint in athletes. This may also be related to numerous problems, but the lack of adequate fat burning due to poor aerobic function is very common. The result is more reliance on sugar for energy—not just during training but at all other times as well.
- **Increased body fat.** This problem is associated with reduced fat burning, causing more fat from dietary carbohydrates and fat to be stored.
- **Chronic inflammation** is one result of higher body fat. Chronic inflammation can also trigger certain injuries and ill health.
- **Physical injuries.** These are often the result of poor aerobic muscle function because these muscles support our joints, bone, ligaments, and other structures. Clinical observations reveal the most common areas of injury in athletes with ADS include the low back, knee, ankle, and foot.
- **Hormonal imbalance.** This common problem interferes with many aspects of fitness and health. It is often associated with high levels of cortisol and low amounts of DHEA. High cortisol may trigger insomnia, high body fat, craving for sweets, and blood sugar irregularities, all with the potential to interfere with proper recovery. Low DHEA can result in low testosterone and other hormones. In women, premenstrual syndrome and menopausal symptoms may be complaints, and in men, low testosterone can adversely affect muscles and bones. Loss of normal sexual

function can affect both men and women as a result of reduced sex hormones.

- **Reduced endurance.** This is often seen with increasing fatigue, poor performance, loss of aerobic speed, and, in general, over-training.
- **Nutritional imbalance.** Dietary problems are often associated with ADS, especially in athletes who consume excess refined carbohydrates and have low fat and protein intakes. Other nutritional imbalances may also occur, such as low iron levels, which adversely affect the "red" iron-dependent aerobic muscles. In addition, the vitamin folate, is an essential nutrient for the aerobic system (necessary for red blood cells to carry oxygen). But many athletes don't get enough because of a genetic mutation. Vitamin D is another important nutrient deficiency surprisingly seen in athletes. (Folate and vitamin D are addressed in more detail later in the book.)

Correction of ADS is relatively easy: build a great aerobic base. One often-neglected factor is choosing the wrong training heart rate.

Do Heart Rate Formulas Work?

Building the aerobic system involves a specific period of sub-max training. While most athletes can no longer train by intuition (which may be due to trends such as no pain no gain, and other social influences), the use of heart rate adds an important component of objectivity, both for training and testing. Heart rate monitors make this very practical.

But which heart rate should be used? There are many ideas about finding the best training heart rates. In one sense, it may not matter, as long as it is associated with a sub-max level of intensity, and that progress is being made with a relatively objective and regular evaluation. Otherwise, training becomes a guessing game.

Most athletes are familiar with the many heart rate formulas out there that supposedly guide you to better training. Perhaps the oldest, and one still around despite little to no scientific rationale, is the 220 Formula. What makes this and the various similar versions obsolete is that they rely on obtaining a maximum heart rate.

The Myth of Max Heart Rates

The maximum heart rate is sometimes determined following hard physical activity, such as running as fast as possible to exhaustion on a track, or a graded test on a treadmill. The highest heart rate is recorded at the end of the run. This approach is most accurate when performed in a controlled condition in a laboratory. Even this approach is not optimal as maximum heart rates may still vary within a given athlete on a given day.

The maximum heart rate is frequently estimated by formula. These are two popular methods:

- By subtracting one's age from 220 (220 minus age). This may overestimate the maximum heart rate when compared to the more accurately measured rate in a laboratory, and can increase the risk of overtraining.
- A second formula sometimes used is 208 minus 0.7 times age. This may underestimate the maximum heart rate when compared to the more accurately measured rate in a laboratory, and may result in a loss of optimal fitness.

It's not unusual for maximum heart rates, especially when measured by a formula, to be significantly off—too high or too low. Without an accurate maximum heart rate, the formulas that require this number become inaccurate as well.

Other factors associated with maximum heart rates include:

- Maximum heart rates vary between different types of activities. Running would produce the highest maximum rate compared to cycling or swimming in the same person. This is due to the increased amount of muscle mass associated with more gravitational stress that accompanies running compared to other activities.

- Maximum heart rate may also vary due to a person's training and stress levels (level of rest), nutritional status (such as hydration), weather (high versus low humidity), and other factors. This can produce a wide variety of maximum heart rates; a group of forty-year old athletes can have a normal range of maximum heart rates between 160 to 200 beats per minute.

- The maximum heart rate can change with training. In particular, the maximum rate can decrease with successful aerobic training. This is due to increased efficiency of the heart, changes in blood volume and other factors. It's also been shown that maximum heart rate can increase during periods of reduced training. These variations can be about 5 percent.

The best recommendations: Avoid formulas that rely on maximum heart rates as part of the equation.

How is maximum heart rate useful for those who work out? While many athletes talk about their levels, often believing that higher is better, which is not necessarily true, there are at least two uses of maximum heart rate.

- I recommend using a percent of maximum heart rate to obtain a general guideline for training during anaerobic work. This may be the training intensity that produces maximum benefits, and rising above this heart rate during an anaerobic workout may produce little or no additional benefits while adding potentially harmful stress. This is 90 percent of your maximum heart rate. It's useful during interval training, hill repeats, and any anaerobic workout except weight lifting (where monitoring the heart rate is much less important).

- Another use of maximum heart rate is to compare your rate as determined in training to a general formula that predicts max heart rate. Athletes who don't come reasonably close to their predicted maximum heart rate, compared to the actual one determined during a hard workout, could have a problem with the nervous system (specifically, the autonomic nervous system) which controls the heart, blood vessels, and other areas—and can even indicate an increased risk of sudden death (these cases are sometimes associated with very low maximum heart rates).

Are Women's Heart Rates Lower than Men's?

A recent study by Dr. Martha Gulati and her colleagues from Northwestern University was published in the medical journal *Circulation*. They measured heart rate responses to exercise stress tests in 5,437 women (average age fifty-two). After a sixteen-year follow up (in which about 549 women—a very high and an alarming 10 percent—died of various causes), the researchers found an important association between the maximum exercise heart rates and age, and they determined a better max heart-rate formula for women undergoing stress tests to help predict those at higher health risk.

But the media, as is often the case with newly published medical studies, have leaped to a number of misleading conclusions. Foremost is this: women who exercise now have a new max heart-rate formula. But the formula determined by this study does not definitively show a woman's maximum heart rate; it's only an estimate. The study also does not replace the old 220 Formula, since this formula has been shown to be inaccurate in determining maximum heart rate in both men and women. Finally, the Northwestern study and the formula do not provide any new information about the best exercise heart rate for woman.

While the study was important because it provides more information on women and heart disease, the subjects of this study were not necessarily athletes. In fact, most were overweight and overfat, and many had high cholesterol and blood pressure, and some were smokers.

The "new female" formula these researchers determined is 206 minus 88 percent of age. But this provides only a general estimate of the peak heart rate a healthy woman should attain during exercise stress tests, and not during regular exercise. The study does not compare or highlight other factors that may be as or more useful in determining increased risk of heart disease, including heart-rate variability, waist circumference, blood pressure, and family/personal health history.

Rather than a formula that relies on one's maximum heart rate, other approaches can be used to help find an optimal aerobic max training heart rate. In a clinical setting, one can determine the respiratory quotient, noted above, which reveals the amount of fat and sugar burned at various heart rates. This may be the basis for determining an effective max aerobic heart rate.

(The VO_{2max} test is popular, and obtaining the respiratory quotient is sometimes done during the same evaluation. But more scientists, clinicians, and coaches have criticized VO_{2max} as not being a valid measure of performance prediction.)

The 180 Formula

By the later 1970s, I began determining the maximum aerobic training heart rates for athletes through clinical evaluations. These included an assessment of various health and fitness factors, gait analysis, and MAF tests. In order to find an easy-to-use formula for athletes that also incorporated age, health, and fitness factors, I developed a formula that did not require knowing the maximum heart rate. It would become known as the 180-formula (see Appendix A). Subsequent RQ and other studies published by others, and consistent progress by athletes in virtually all sports using the formula since the early 1980s, has helped further support to the usefulness of the 180 Formula.

While the 180 Formula was developed from careful clinical research, it is not the perfect formula either. However, it appears to be the most successful one available.

The Ultimate Sub-Max Test

Whether running, biking, skiing, or performing other endurance training, measuring ones maximum aerobic function is easy to do. It may be the best endurance test for all athletes to monitor their aerobic systems, and a way to measure progress, helping to take the guesswork out of training.

This is easily accomplished by running, biking, or using any endurance activity at one's sub-max training heart rate. I prefer using the 180 Formula.

The maximum aerobic function (MAF) test was developed in conjunction with the 180 Formula as a way to help confirm that the training heart rate and base building is progressing well. (Appendix B summarizes the MAF Test.)

Any program, regardless of its philosophy, can be measured with the MAF Test. In short, if you are truly progressing, you'll be able to run, bike or swim faster at the same submaximal heart rate as the months pass. If you observe this important aspect of training, it also means your body is burning more fat, health is improving with less injury and illness, there is typically some weight loss, and better race results will follow.

Why I No Longer Like Lactate Testing

Blood lactate, which comes from lactic acid production in all muscles, is an important fuel for the body rather than the dead-end waste product many think it to be. Even at rest, lactate is being produced in small amounts.

This important compound is used for energy throughout the body, especially in the heart, brain, liver, and by the muscles themselves. And lactate has also been shown to contribute directly to glycogen synthesis in our muscles and liver.

When working out, we rely on lactate as an important source of glucose, even on an easy run. For example, when burning fat and sugar for energy, the total amount of sugar comes from three main sources:

- A smaller amount comes from the glucose in the blood.
- A varying amount comes from glycogen (stored glucose in muscle) and a moderate amount comes from lactate. Total CHO oxidation is the summed use of blood lactate, blood glucose, and muscle glycogen.
- Blood lactate can be considered a primary source of sugar and, as such, capable of delaying the depletion of glycogen stores during competition.
- These are some of the reasons to like lactate. Measuring it is another story.

Evaluating Lactate

When I started working with athletes in 1977, measuring an individual's many health and fitness features was a priority. My education emphasized this process, and the experience quickly taught me how important it would be in uncovering the cause of an injury and other problems that interfered with athletic progress.

Evaluations included treadmill and cycling testing in my clinic, and field evaluations on the track, in the pool, and at other locations. From samples of blood, urine, and saliva, more assessments meant additional data to better fine-tune the athlete. Specific tests included lactate, along with hormones, fats, vitamins, minerals, enzymes, red and white blood cells, and many others. In addition, analysis of posture and gait, and biofeedback assessments including muscle testing were important. An ongoing oral health and fitness history may have been the most important assessment tool, which is still true today.

This process took considerable time. As the years passed I reduced the use of those tests that provided less information—especially the ones that told me what other more useful evaluations provided. Low on the list was blood lactate.

Today's technology allows easy and accurate measurement of lactate. Traditionally tested from blood, other high-tech tests will hit the market soon. For example, a new biosensor in the form of a temporary tattoo is being developed that will measure lactate in sweat.

There are several reasons I stopped testing lactate. Training lactate levels do not reflect production from lactic acid in muscles but, rather its clearance from the blood. This might appear academic, but those who metabolize it quicker have lower levels, while others may maintain higher ones. The ability to break down lactate is a reflection of overall health, in particular that of the liver and kidneys, with the nutritional status being particularly important. All these factors can change from day to day, and even within a single day.

While there is a significant difference between lactate levels in trained and untrained individuals, the state of one's fitness is also an important factor. Varying levels of both aerobic and anaerobic fitness influence the amount of lactate in the blood. So the concept that there is a particular "point" or threshold is very misleading—this may be the case on a given day or month, but it will change. Relying on a single lactate number—even a series of them over the course of a week or month—becomes potentially misleading. (Also know that scientists consider various factors associated with lactate: anaerobic threshold, lactate threshold, onset of blood lactate accumulation, onset of plasma lactate accumulation, heart rate deflection point, and maximum lactate steady state.)

Various lifestyle factors can influence lactate, including the diet. Thiamin (vitamin B1) and magnesium are examples of two key nutritional substances found in a healthy diet that are necessary in sufficient amounts to properly metabolize lactate. Lower levels of these nutrients are associated with higher lactate readings, with the real possibility of misinterpretation and other errors when applying the results to training.

A computerized diet analysis, which I used throughout my career, is still an excellent, easy, and inexpensive way to assess one's nutrient intake. In large numbers of athletes, thiamin and magnesium (and often other nutrients) do not even reach minimum RDA levels, a reflection of poor eating. In addition to lactate, this will have negative effects on other areas of athletic function. (The answer to this problem is not supplementation but improving the overall quality of food consumption.)

I also no longer recommend lactate testing because there are more-reliable, easier, and cheaper evaluations that all athletes can regularly utilize for effective training. Included is the MAF test.

Beware: The New *No Pain No Gain* Trend

Is Aerobic Exercise Bad?

As much as it pains me to restate the obvious, "no pain no gain" is an outdated, unhealthy obsession that is regrettably back in the news. Online forums, articles, and even books now percolate with the mistaken belief that aerobic training is bad and harmful. It's like saying the world is flat or the sky is falling. Perhaps someone should add, *Throw away your heart monitor and brain and just do it!*

I say don't just do it—do it right!

Is aerobic exercise really bad for us? Does it shrink our heart and lungs, and cause muscle wasting, like proponents say? No. The magic of marketing misinformation is a monster that's replaced logic in the new world order of high tech. It's an extension of the misleading advertising styles that began in the early days of television, when doctors told us cigarettes were healthy and Wonder Bread built strong bodies twelve ways. (Both are examples of ads forced off the air by the Federal Trade Commission because they were false.)

Unfortunately, when it comes to exercise, anyone can say anything, not matter how absurd or cultish.

It was just a matter of time when the *harder-is-better* folk would usher in a new, but not improved, era of the "no pain no gain" philosophy. This time they're fighting back hard. They are doing it by trashing the other side, a common marketing and political ploy. And they even succeeded in turning it into quite a debate. But I'm not jumping on this bandwagon—there are too many other intelligent facts to read and write about. But I will make a few comments.

"Should I train slow or fast?" I'm asked. "Aerobic or anaerobic?" "Lift weights or walk?" The correct answer, of course, is an easy one—do it all! Balance and individualization are very important.

What's even more laughable is that the no pain no gainers claim there's no evidence that aerobic exercise is healthy. Really? Tens of thousands of published studies clearly demonstrate that aerobic training offers untold number of benefits, and without harmful side effects.

There will always be unscrupulous people who twist information to get something they want. Take the tobacco companies— they still don't believe enough research shows cigarette smoking is harmful. Guess we need to spend millions more on additional studies (which is actually still being done).

Eat more vegetables and fruits for added health? More research is needed—and millions of dollars are being spent to do just that too.

Oh, by the way, many of those millions come from our tax dollars. And much of it is wasted. A recent *British Medical Journal* report states that the information from many drug studies, for example, is being suppressed by researchers because the outcome is not what they wanted. In fact, less than half of the studies paid for by the U.S. National Institutes for Health were not published. (The NIH spends about $3.5 billion annually for research.)

Among the problems with the new, modern "no pain no gain" approach is the key words being discussed and debated are never defined. Terms such as "aerobic" and "anaerobic" are merely two examples.

Nor do they consider the "health" of an individual, or differentiate this from "fitness." One email I received about the anti-aerobic approach said that endurance training shrinks your heart and lungs. Hmm, doesn't the endurance heart get larger? (Yes, it's referred to as an *athletic heart*.)

Yet another new study (in *The Physician and Sports Medicine*), which included triathletes, runners, and swimmers, demonstrated how long-term endurance training builds and maintains muscle mass and strength very effectively later in life, and prevents excess fat accumulation. (Ho hum, this was shown decades ago.)

When do we stop trying to prove common sense? Two new expensive studies from Harvard were published recently, showing that running in flat shoes and forefoot strikes are less injurious to runners than wearing thick shoes and heel striking. I often receive emails on the *debate* about whether barefoot running is healthy or not. Debate? Haven't humans been doing this successfully for millions of years?

There are also many exercise physiology textbooks, from McGardle & Katch to Wilmore & Costill, that for decades have described the many benefits of aerobic exercise—from the thirty-minute-a-day walker to those training for long endurance events. (These also contain tens of thousands of peer-reviewed indexed studies on the subject.)

Despite this, we still hear how endurance exercise shrinks muscle mass, increases body fat production and stress hormones, impairs immunity, decreases heart reserve, and increases triglyc erides and LDL cholesterol. Well, the fact is, training the aerobic system properly does just the opposite!

Perhaps the new "no pain no gain" crowd is confused because, as is well known, *overtraining* can cause the problems they talk about. But I've read nowhere that it's the caveat they warn people about. Instead, it's aerobic exercise itself that's evil, they say.

If you look at the outcome of even a single bout of easy aerobic versus hard anaerobic activity, it brings the issue into better perspective. Easy aerobic workouts train the body to increase fat burning over the next twenty-four hours, while anaerobic exercise reduces it, instead promoting sugar burning. Aerobic muscle fibers, unlike the anaerobic types are much more extensive in the human body, uniquely support our structure, helping to prevent muscle, joint, ligament, tendon and bone injuries. And a single, short hard workout can significantly increase the stress hormone cortisol, causing significant protein loss through the kidneys (proteinuria), reductions in fat burning, and other metabolic stress—not so with aerobic training.

In addition, as other research clearly shows, *unhealthy* people who exercise—both during aerobic and anaerobic training, and while competing—can die of heart attacks, even when having sex. I wonder when we'll see a book about avoiding sex because it's dangerous to our health?

FAT BURNING CAN SAVE YOUR ENDURANCE WORLD

An important concept I began promoting in the late 1970s is the notion of *"want speed, slow down."* In order to accomplish this feat one must have a healthy metabolism with fat as a dominant fuel. Without this part of the equation, training slow will just result in more slow training because the aerobic system never has enough energy from fat to effectively develop itself.

Many athletes are stuck in the slower mode because of reduced energy. And, many of those who race fast are unable to get faster for the same reason. In order to shift energy sources to increased fat burning, lifestyle must be modified—this includes eating fewer carbohydrate foods to match the training that builds the fat-burning aerobic system. If you want to raise the level of your endurance, you'll need more energy.

Nothing impacts humanity more than the air we breathe and food we consume. These simple essentials generate energy for our brains to think and bodies to act. But not only energy for idle thought and simple movement; also energy to endure as a species, and for better training and racing.

Energy is enabling, it's our life force. It propelled the earliest humans to evolve with amazing mental and physical promise. That potential is still with us today.

When we talk about the body's use of energy, we are, of course, referring to the calorie. But one must ask, "Calories of what?" The answer is that we commonly burn a mix of fat and sugar calories.

Right now, we are all fueling our bodies with a certain balance of fat and sugar. Some of us convert more fat for energy, even the leanest among us, while others less so. If we don't burn enough fat calories, they remain stored as body fat, and we increase reliance on sugar for fuel, which, as discuss in the last section of this book, is very limited.

With limited energy, life is impaired. Our brains and bodies don't function as well. Evolution turns its other cheek.

Energy restriction in a single person can cause poor health and reduced fitness; in a family, disharmony; for a population, society weakens; and in the masses, it can impair our planet.

There is now a worldwide epidemic of billions of people with poor fat burning and low energy. The obesity plague is proof of that, but it's only the tip of the iceberg. Many more people are "overfat"—a better term that defines this physiological problem—despite society dancing around the "f" word, trying to be politically correct. Fat is not a four-letter word.

The majority of the world's population is now overfat—those who burn too little causing it to accumulate throughout the body, even in people who are not technically obese.

The problem is not limited to industrialized societies. It even affects third-world countries where, in the course of a single generation, the obesity epidemic has outpaced starvation—the World Health Organization calls this the *Nutrition Transition*.

No doubt some of us remember when there were very few overweight students in our 1950s grade-school classes. Today, childhood obesity is skyrocketing.

To make matters worse, the overfat epidemic has not spared athletes.

As endurance animals, we require continuous, untiring energy, even while sleeping. Increased fat burning makes us healthier, we think better, and are more fit. Otherwise, we are biologically impaired.

While we can feel poor fat burning as low energy, we can see its deadly outcome on a larger scale. Witness the crippling economies unable to keep up with spiraling healthcare costs due to the overfat epidemic, which directly spawns chronic disease—cancer, heart disease, Alzheimer's, diabetes, to name a few. Experts say the worst is coming soon.

We can measure an individual's fat and sugar burning in a laboratory or clinic, while on a bike, running or walking on a treadmill, or at rest. But this is not usually necessary—most people already know when they're not burning enough body fat. Low energy, health issues, fitness not progressing, and clothes fitting too tight are common indicators.

There are two common reasons for poor fat burning.

The first is junk food.

There are two basic cuisines on our planet today—healthy food and junk food. Healthy food is real, and includes such items as fresh vegetables and fruits, raw nuts and seeds, real meat and cheese, and whole eggs. Junk food is processed, and its main ingredient is refined carbohydrate. This includes sugar in all its forms, and flour, even if it's called whole grain, which quickly turns to sugar after we eat it.

Many people don't realize that a lot of junk food is well-disguised and made to appear healthy. Much of it is even found in health stores. One example is organic junk food—something to also avoid.

Refined carbohydrates are everywhere: in cereals, bagels, breads, muffins, energy bars, sports drinks, snacks, packaged foods, pasta, and many others. When going through this list with patients, they would usually stop me at some point and say, "That's all I eat!" I would say, "*That* is why you're here."

In the time it takes to eat even a small junk food snack or even a big bite—we can swing our metabolism from high-energy fat burning to low energy fat storing. We often feel this right after a meal—mental fatigue, reduced concentration, or even sleepiness.

This occurs because a higher amount of the hormone insulin is produced when we consume refined carbs. This does two things to our bodies. First, it converts up to half the carbs we eat into stored fat; and second, at the same time, reduces our ability to burn high amounts of body fat.

Eating refined carbs can also trigger cravings for more sweets. This maintains a vicious cycle simply called sugar addiction. The junk food industry has created a world of sugar junkies, and perhaps worse than what big tobacco has done.

The remedy: don't eat any junk food, starting right now! To make sure you understand what junk food really is, further descriptions of junk food can be found in Section 7.

A second cause of the overfat epidemic is related to physical activity. This is all about balance. As discussed in the previous section, each workout immediately influences fat and sugar burning. As we all know, not enough physical activity contributes to being overfat. But on the other extreme, so can overtraining, as evident in the many athletes with surprisingly high amounts of body fat, despite working out for 10, 15, 20, or more hours each week. They burn a lot of calories, just too few in the form of fat.

Developing our aerobic systems is how we learn to burn more body fat—unless, of course, the process is impaired by eating junk food.

A recent article in the *European Journal of Sports Science* entitled, "Rethinking fat as a fuel for endurance exercise," reviewed what many have known and implemented for years. It's been the foundation of my method from the beginning, for both improvements in race performance and optimal health. Lead author Jeff Velek states, "A key element contributing to deteriorating exercise capacity during physically demanding sport appears to be reduced carbohydrate availability coupled with an inability to effectively utilize alternative lipid [fat] fuel sources."

Read a real case history, below.

"Why Am I Overfat—I Burn So Many Calories?"

While the world is now in the midst of a serious overfat epidemic, surprisingly athletes have not been spared. Here is one case.

A patient of mine many years ago, PT (not the real initials), enjoyed running but didn't complain about the slow-race pace. In our initial meeting, PT did not mention the chronic knee problem, the off and on hip pain that would occasionally prevent training, or the fatigue that had been worsening in recent years. Averaging more than fifty-five miles a week of running, sometime over sixty miles, PT's lofty goal was to run a marathon, having barely struggled to the finish of three 13.1-mile efforts.

One of PT's main complaints was too much body fat. A dietary analysis seemed to make no sense—enough calories were being burned from running, without an excess in the diet. In fact, PT claimed to be a careful eater, keeping clear of fatty foods and snacks. Hunger, however, was a frequent problem.

There are possibly millions of athletes like PT. They run, bike, sweat for untold numbers of workout hours in gyms, aerobics classes, and with home exercise DVDs. And they watch what they eat. But clearly, something is wrong in many of these individuals. Body fat keeps rising. These would-be and want-to-be lean athletes have failed in their attempt to accomplish what others seem to have—both a fit and healthy body without excess fat. Why is it so difficult?

It's not. PT and so many other men and women—young, middle-aged, and older—have metabolisms that could work perfectly normal, but don't. That's because their workouts and the foods consumed are giving the body the wrong signals.

They're programming their bodies to burn more sugar, and less fat. The result? All day, and all night, their body's metabolic engine keeps storing more body fat.

I explained to PT that there are two reasons for this problem. First, the training routine is too hard. Many people think that working out harder will burn more calories. It will, but calories of what? If this is sugar, the body does not train to be a fat burner.

By working out too hard, we teach our body to burn more sugar calories, diminishing fat burning. The result is that our fat stores get bigger.

Sure, this is contrary to most magazine articles and blogs people read every day; and it was quite different to basically everything PT's training friends were talking about. Many of them were overfat, too. "Please just tell me what to do," PT said and apologized for interrupting me—her years of frustration being obvious.

The remedy: Slow down. I told PT to consider the total number of minutes she worked out, not miles, and to maintain that schedule. Running slower with a lower heart rate would help retrain the body to burn more fat—not just during the workout, but twenty-four hours a day. Yes, even during sleep.

Second, the foods we eat influence the burning of sugar and fat, even more than training.

I explained to PT that some people burn more fat and less sugar even at rest. They are leaner, less injured, perform better, and are healthier. Others, who may even consume the same number of calories, burn more sugar and much less fat. The result? You guessed it—they store more body fat.

Why is this? As more thoroughly discussed in *The Big Book of Endurance Training and Racing*, it's the hormone insulin.

Insulin is produced by the pancreas each time we eat carbohydrate foods—particularly the refined and low-fat variety. The more carbs, the more insulin.

Insulin takes the carbohydrates we eat, which quickly become glucose in the blood, and uses some of it for immediate energy. Insulin stores a small amount of glucose for later use, but 40 to 50 percent of the carbohydrate we eat turn to stored fat. If we don't burn it, there it remains.

I explained this important mechanism to PT, who seemed dazed. "What should I eat?" she asked, desperately seeking answers.

The remedy is simple. Avoid refined carbohydrates.

Refined carbs cause us to store more body fat. This includes processed wheat products including virtually all breads, rolls, muffins, pancakes, and cereals, along with potatoes and corn, including chips; all sweets do the same. In addition, so-called energy bars and sports drinks are big culprits, and products containing hidden sugars such as ketchup, salad dressing, and a surprising number of packaged, canned, and bottled foods must be avoided.

"That's all I eat," PT said and sat up, anxiously. "But they're all low fat."

"And half of these low-fat foods turn to stored body fat," I emphasized. "They stimulate insulin, triggering a significant amount of those carbs to be stored as fat in the hips, thigh, buttocks, belly, arms—everywhere."

To make things even worse, insulin also reduces the body's ability to burn fat, *even with the right training schedule*. So diet really oversees our training body.

Fresh fruit, lentils, beans, and even small amounts of honey can be part of a healthy diet that helps reduce body fat because these healthy carbs trigger less insulin.

PT surrendered, reluctantly agreeing to eliminate refined carbohydrates, including all sugar from the diet. It would be replaced by fresh fruits and vegetables, eggs for breakfast instead of cereal, meat or fish as part of a healthy lunch and dinner, and snacking on almonds, cashews, and a variety of other healthy food items when hungry—foods that would not impair fat-burning.

After two weeks of training slower, and avoiding all refined carbohydrates, PT's energy improved, the mechanical injuries nearly disappeared, and for the first time in several years, PT lost weight—six pounds! After another two weeks, five more pounds.

It would not be long before PT's clothes were fitting looser. People even began asking if PT was feeling okay.

Gradually, PT could consume some natural carbohydrates, but maintained a strict avoidance of refined foods, especially sugar. She learned how to make healthy desserts, and now PT never gets hungry and began feeling younger. About three months later, PT needed to buy new clothes to fit the now-leaner body. And, after another few months, passing dozens of runners in the last two miles of a successful marathon was a joy for her to experience.

This section of the book is one that too many endurance athletes skip over or otherwise are not serious about when it comes to making the appropriate dietary changes.

The notion that we can lose weight *and* those extra inches, improve performance, and get healthier all at the same time is quite real. It's a package deal, so to speak. It is as simple as adjusting our metabolism to promote more fat burning. And there's no long wait—the process begins the very first day of making the necessary changes.

To meet our body's continuous energy demand, we burn calories all day and night. More specifically, our metabolism converts both sugar and fat into ATP, a primary source of energy. Those individuals who burn more fat calories, and fewer sugar calories, are healthier with less injuries and illness, and have higher physical energy. They also have less stored body fat, and usually are close to their optimal weight. For athletes, burning more body fat is the secret to improved performance. Below is an example of how increased fat burning improves racing.

Walter Burns Fat to 7th World Championship

July 2013: Hal Walter wins the 29-mile World Championship Pack-Burro Race in Colorado with a jenny named Full Tilt Boogie, using training and nutrition methods he's learned from Dr. Phil Maffetone over the past fifteen years. For more than five hours of rigorous racing, Walter relied on water only, and his stored body fat for fuel.

Walter was Phil's editor from 1998 to 2004, working with him on several books, the Maffetone Report newsletter and other projects.

The annual event is held on a rugged mountainous course from the town of Fairplay, elevation 10,000 feet, to the top of 13,187-foot Mosquito Pass and back. Competitors run and hike the steeper pitches with their burros but may not ride. The animals carry 33-pound packs, including a pick, pan and shovel to commemorate the state's mining history.

Walter says the race is much more demanding than a typical marathon or triathlon due to the extremes in elevation, vertical gain, weather conditions and terrain, not to mention managing an animal not known for its cooperative nature. He's also competed in marathons, ultramarathons and winter multi-sport competitions.

Walter attributes his success to a high degree of fat-burning achieved over the years of training using aerobic training and a diet customized to suit his needs. He notes that he drank only water and ate nothing during the entire event, which Dr. Maffetone says is an indication of an excellent fat-burning capacity.

Walter also notes he does very little anaerobic training, but this did not keep him from having a finishing kick.

The race boiled down to a contest between Walter and Boogie, and George Zack of Broomfield and his burro Jack. The teams traded places as many as 30 times over the course of the race, with Walter and Boogie finally pulling ahead near the finish line, winning in five hours, twenty-five minutes and twenty-three seconds. Zack and Jack, who won the race last year, finished only two seconds behind.

"In the last few steps her ears went forward and she made a gallant charge," said Walter. "It was all heart and it was all Boogie. Luckily I had the legs to go with her."

This is Walter's seventh world championship in fifteen years and, at fifty-three, it is believed he is the oldest person to win in the sixty-five-year history of the event.

There are two primary factors that influence our ability to increase fat burning: eating healthy, unrefined foods; and working out easier rather than harder.

Eating Healthy Foods

Our diet plays a key role in dictating how much fat burning takes place. Certain foods encourage the process while others impair it. Generally speaking, refined carbohydrates, including sugar, flour, and other processed foods, immediately reduce fat burning when eaten. To make things worse, up to half of these unhealthy foods are immediately converted to stored fat. Because the body is unable to burn as much fat calories, they are stored.

Healthy foods including fresh fruits and vegetables, protein foods (meat, fish, eggs, cheese), nuts, and seeds can help promote fat burning.

Be careful with food selection as many packaged foods—perhaps most—contain hidden sugars. This is also true for many restaurant items.

Food Frequency

Another important way to improve metabolism is to increase food frequency. Gone are the days when dieting meant hunger and cravings. By eating more frequent healthy meals, snacks, and even desserts, the process of increased fat burning continues unimpeded. For most individuals with too much body fat, eating something healthy every two to four hours is important to stimulate the burning of more body fat.

Why We Just Can't Stop Eating Sugar

This is an easy question to answer: sugar is addictive. Obviously it is, otherwise billions of people would not be overeating it.

A Simple Body Fat Test: Measure Your Waist

The most simple and practical way to calculate changes in body fat is to periodically measure your waist with a tape measure at the level of the umbilicus, or the belly button. Most people already know this, as increasing levels of body fat result in clothes fitting tighter, especially around the waist. Likewise when burning off more body fat, it's often recognized when clothes become looser.

Unfortunately, you can't dictate where fat loss occurs first. Nor can you spot reduce by doing countless sit-ups or crunches. The belly fat won't burn off that way. But as you burn more body fat, you will notice that your clothes are fitting loosely. People will also tell you that you look thinner, often noticing it first in your face. Since bathroom scale weight is mostly a measure of water, the measurement of fat, which is what most of us need to know, can't be determined accurately on the scale. It's not unusual, for example, for a person to gain body fat as reflected in a larger waist size, but show no weight gain on the scale. Likewise, it's not unusual to lose a couple of inches on your waist and not lose weight.

Body Fat: The Good, Bad, and Ugly

When it comes to body fat, there are two kinds—good and bad. When bad fat takes over the body, it's ugly. When talking about obtaining energy by burning body fat, I am obviously referring to good fat— even a lean person has enough stored fat to run hundreds, even thousands, of miles. When it comes to the diet, the trend continues to be the myth that less is best.

The Big Fat Food Lie

When it comes to fatty foods, this has been seen as the "bad" component of our diet. Low- and no-fat has become synonymous with being healthy. These ideas, of course, are untrue. In fact, fat is one of the most beneficial substances in your diet, and is often the missing ingredient in developing and maintaining optimal health and human performance. But an ongoing, well-financed misinformation campaign against fat has misled the public to an epidemic of fat phobia. Just think of the billions of dollars spent each year on low-fat and fat-free foods and you'll understand why you might not have been told the whole truth about fat. In addition, this anti-fat campaign has contributed to actual deficiencies in fat that have contributed to various diseases. The bottom line on dietary fat: too much or too little is dangerous. It's simply a question of balancing your intake.

First, let's define fat—a term that also includes oil. Fats are found in concentrated forms such as vegetable oils, butter, egg yolk, cheeses, and other naturally occurring foods, and in less concentrated forms that make up the content of almost all natural foods. And some foods contain very small fat components that are as essential as all other nutrients.

Virtually all natural fats are healthy. As noted above, eating a balance of fats is most important. This issue is discussed in more detail in the next two chapters. In general, eating too much of one type of fat, such as too much saturated fat from dairy products or too much omega-6 fat from vegetable oil, is an example of a fat imbalance that can adversely affect health. In addition, eating "bad" fat—those that are artificial and highly processed, such as trans fat and overheated fats in fried foods—can cause serious health problems. Foods such as chips, French fries, and fried chicken, to name just a few, are examples of those containing bad fat.

Dietary fats have been a staple for humans throughout evolution. Ironically many people are learning of the true importance of fats in the diet only through the low-fat trend of the last few decades. This is not news, really. Scientists have known of the importance of fat in the diet since the discoveries in 1929 by researchers who demonstrated the necessity of dietary fat.

When it comes to stored body fat, there are still many good, healthy features we should know about in addition to the generation of energy from stored fat. Here are some of them:

- **Hormones.** The hormonal system is responsible for controlling virtually all healthy functions of the body. But for this system to function properly, the body must produce proper amounts of the appropriate hormones. These are produced in various glands, dependent on fat for production of hormones. The adrenal glands, the thymus, thyroid, kidneys, and other glands use fats to help make hormones. Cholesterol is one of the fats used for the production of hormones such as progesterone and cortisone. The thymus gland regulates immunity and the body's defense systems. The thyroid regulates temperature, weight, and other metabolic functions. The kidney's hormones help regulate blood pressure, circulation, and filtering of blood. Some hormonal problems are associated with body-fat content that's too low. For example, some women with very low body fat, from too much exercise or very poor diet habits, experience disruptions in their menstrual cycle. In older women, this may also effect menopausal symptoms.

- **Insulation.** The body's ability to store fat permits humans to live in most climates, particularly in areas of extreme heat or cold. In warmer areas of the world, stored fat provides protection from the heat. In colder lands, increased fat stored beneath the skin prevents too much heat from leaving the body. An example of fat's effectiveness as an insulator is in an Eskimo's ability to withstand great cold and survive in good health. Eskimos eat a high fat diet, and despite this have very low incidence of heart disease and other ailments. In warmer climates, fat prevents too much water from leaving the body, which can result in dehydration that causes dry, scaly skin. Some evaporation is normal, of course, but fats under the skin regulate evaporation and can prevent as much as ten to twenty times more water from leaving the body.

- **Healthy Skin and Hair.** Fat has protective qualities that also give skin the soft, smooth, and unwrinkled appearance that many people try to achieve through expensive skin conditioners. The healthy look of skin comes from the fat inside. The same is true for your hair. Fats, including cholesterol, also serve as an insulating barrier within the skin. Without this protection, water and water-soluble substances such as chemical pollutants would enter the body through the skin. With the proper balance and amounts of fats in your diet, your skin and hair develop a healthy appearance. If you've been looking for the ideal skin and hair product, you can have it by balancing the fats in your diet.

- **Support and Protection.** Stored fat offers physical support and protection to vital body parts, including the organs and glands. Fat acts as a natural, built-in shock absorber, cushioning the body and its various parts from the wear and tear of everyday life, and helps prevent organs from sinking due to the downward pull of gravity. Fats also may protect the body against the harmful effects of X-rays. This occurs through physical protection of the cell, and by controlling free-radical production, generated as a result of X-ray exposure. In addition to medical X-rays, we are constantly exposed to X-rays from the atmosphere. This cosmic radiation penetrates most objects, including airplanes. The average person gets more cosmic radiation exposure during an airline flight from New York to Los Angeles than from a lifetime of medical X-rays.

- **Vitamin and Mineral Regulation.** Most people know that vitamin D is produced by exposure of the skin to the sun. However, it is actually cholesterol in the skin that allows this reaction to occur. Sunlight chemically changes cholesterol in the skin through the process of irradiation to vitamin D-3. This newly formed vitamin D is then absorbed into the blood, allowing calcium and phosphorous to be properly absorbed from the intestinal tract. Without the vitamin D, calcium and phosphorous would not be well absorbed and deficiencies of both could occur. But without cholesterol, the entire process would not occur. Besides vitamin D, other vitamins, including A, E, and K, rely on fat for proper absorption and utilization. These important vitamins are present primarily in fatty foods, and the body cannot make an adequate amount of these vitamins to ensure continued good health. In addition these vitamins require fat in the intestines in order to be absorbed. So a low-fat diet could be deficient in these vitamins to begin with and also could further restrict their absorption.

Two Types of Body Fat

The human body possesses two distinct types of body fat, referred to as *brown* and *white*. Both forms of body fat are active, living parts of us, heavily influencing our metabolism, protecting our organs, glands and bones, and offering many other health benefits mostly from our stores of white fat. This body fat content ranges from 5 percent in male athletes to more than 50 percent of total body weight in obese individuals. Brown fat makes up only about 1 percent of the total body fat in healthy adults, although it's much more abundant at birth in healthy babies.

Brown fat helps us burn white fat; this is an important aspect of overall health. (Even in athletes, it's an important energy source for better performance.) Without adequate brown fat, we can gain body fat and become sluggish in the winter like a hibernating animal. There are a number of ways to increase brown fat activity.

Certain foods can stimulate brown fat and increase overall fat-burning. Eating several times a day, five to six smaller healthy meals instead of one, two, or three larger ones, for example, can trigger a process called *thermogenesis*—an important post-meal metabolic stimulation for fat-burning. However, if our caloric intake is too low, brown fat can slow the burning of white fat. This can happen on a low-calorie diet and when we skip meals.

Brown fat can be stimulated by certain dietary fats. While omega-3 fats are especially potent, most natural fats, including coconut oil, dairy fat, and extra virgin olive oil can stimulate the body's brown fat.

Other foods that increase brown fat activity include caffeine, but only if it's tolerated. Tea, coffee, and chocolate contain small to high amounts of caffeine. However, if under stress, our adrenal glands become overworked, which can promote fat storage and reduce fat burning; caffeine may worsen adrenal stress in many individuals. Also, avoid coffee, tea, and chocolate products if they contain sugar, which can reduce fat-burning.

Brown fat is greatly controlled by skin temperature. If we get too hot during the day, or overdress during exercise, brown-fat activity can lead to less burning of white fat. This is why wearing extra clothes or "sweatsuits" during exercise, a common weight-loss myth, can be dangerous.

Even sitting in a hot tub, sauna, or steam room regularly after exercise may offset some of the fat-burning benefits of physical activity. These activities can increase sweating, resulting in some water-weight loss, but the sacrifice is actually less fat-burning. Hot tubs and saunas do come with health benefits, but to avoid the reductions in fat-burning take a minute or two to cool the body in a cold shower or tub afterwards.

In contrast, brown fat is stimulated by cold. Cooling the body's brown-fat areas can help stimulate fat burning. Brown fat is found around the shoulders and underarms, between the ribs and at the nape of the neck. These are important areas to keep from over-heating and to cool after exercise.

Unfortunately, most research in the area of brown fat comes from the pharmaceutical industry, which is looking for a new drug to stimulate brown fat. But a healthy diet, building a great aerobic system, and other lifestyle habits already can do this!

Belly Fat

Call it a beer belly, gut, love handles, or just a bulging waist. Too much stored fat is worse than it looks. Excess abdominal belly fat in particular is a sign of reduced health and lowered fitness. Sadly, the problem has become so common that many young people think it's fashionable. But it's not healthy.

Clinically, a high amount of abdominal fat is called *central obesity*. But one need not be obese—with a worldwide overfat epidemic, no one is exempt from this dilemma, including athletes.

Many people measure body fat with calipers, water weighing, and the latest modern high-tech methods that estimate percent body fat. All are still estimations. While better than pinching the skin or looking in the mirror, which certainly has some value, measuring your waist once a month is a simple way to regularly assess belly fat changes. Of course, most people already know this by how their pants fit.

The Carbo Belly

Getting rid of belly fat has become an obsession for millions of people. While "spot reducing," such as endless sit-ups and crunches, or the latest ab machines to lose belly fat, is a popular trend in gyms everywhere, these approaches are never truly successful because the problem is metabolic, not caused by poor muscle tone. To burn off excess central body fat, the cause of the problem must first be addressed.

Perhaps the most common cause of excess central body fat is refined carbohydrate consumption. Bread, cereal, pasta, potatoes, sports drinks and bars, and sugar, whether straight or hidden (or obvious) in many packaged products, are among the foods that are high glycemic and the Number One culprit. When consumed, they cause a higher production of insulin, the hormone that converts up to half the carbohydrates one consumes into stored fat, typically in the belly. Insulin also impairs the ability of the body to burn its stored fat for energy.

It's simple: if you want to reduce belly fat, don't eat any more refined carbohydrates! I'm betting most people reading this already know about this most common of health recommendations.

Easier said than done? Possibly. Sugar and other refined carbs are powerfully addictive substances, so just saying no only works for those with a strong brain (will power). But another problem is sugar adversely effects the brain—and that's the vicious cycle.

Increased belly fat is a serious sign of bodywide poor health. It's commonly associated with heart disease, Alzheimer's, cancer, diabetes, and chronic inflammation. The problem is also seen in those with chronically high stress hormone, cortisol, and high blood fats (triglycerides), both easy to measure—cortisol in saliva and triglycerides in blood.

Many people work out regularly yet still carry around too much belly fat, despite all the calories burned in training. The problem, of course, is that not enough *fat* calories are used.

In addition to increasing your pants size, increased belly fat can stretch the abdominal muscles. This lengthening causes them to weaken, triggering the sacrospinalis muscles in the back to tighten. This is a common recipe for chronic low back pain and disability. The same problem also alters gait and can interfere with exercise efficiency whether walking, running, biking, swimming, or other activities. For a competitive athlete, this can be devastating.

By being both healthy and fit, and sometimes with the help of an appropriate healthcare professional, correction of these imbalances is possible. The problem of excess abdominal fat is relatively easy to remedy—avoid eating refined carbohydrates.

First Meal-Fat Storage

Breakfast is the most important meal of the day because it replaces lost nutrients in the body used during sleep. Skipping this meal is one of the worst bad nutrition habits because it can contribute to a big belly. It's important to eat soon after wakening, but not by breaking your all-night fast with just any food.

Many of my new patients who did not eat breakfast were the least healthy and least fit. When asked why no breakfast, a common response was because it made them too hungry throughout the day. Those individuals also had more excess belly fat.

A reason for being hungry all day after eating breakfast is the consumption of a high glycemic meal. Whether cereal, a bagel or muffin, toast, or other refined carbohydrate, this eating pattern is a recipe for too much belly fat. Eating healthy meals, and more frequently, can improve metabolism and help the body burn more fat.

These lifestyle adjustments can help reduce belly fat, slim you down all over, and increase energy and brainpower. In addition, the aerobic system will improve too, helping to reduce injuries, and allow you to train and race faster.

As most already know, the reason refined carbohydrates—and even too much of the natural forms (and sometimes too much protein)—convert to stored fat and reduces fat burning has to do with the hormone insulin.

The Insulin Villain

The idea of injecting oneself with a needle is something many people shun, or even fear. "I'll do anything to avoid that," one patient told me emphatically, many years ago. Yet, he could not—*would not*—change eating habits in a way that would prevent his pancreas from burning out. Only a few months later he was injecting insulin every day.

A diagnosis of diabetes is a hard pill to swallow, even for an athlete. While it's a preventable disease, many succumb to using the needle despite insulin's side effects, which are often devastating. Why? Most won't change their diet—nor do they get help from healthcare professionals, the media, or any other influential source despite the solid science.

A surprising number of people are at risk for becoming diabetic and requiring insulin injections. This includes anyone on the spectrum of carbohydrate intolerance, which may be 75 percent or more of the world's population. The sad fact is many people are unwilling to eat in a way that can prevent them from dropping into a diagnosis of diabetes.

Of course, I'm referring to type 2 diabetes. This form is preventable—something that can be accomplished by reducing carbohydrate foods, including the elimination of moderate and high glycemic foods, especially refined sugars and products made from flour. (At least modest amounts of physical activity are important, too.)

But even in those diagnosed with type 2 diabetes, the pancreas still produces some insulin. It may even be enough to avoid medication—but only if the diet is truly healthy and one is physically active.

The so-called acquired form of diabetes, type 1, is very different. It appears as an autoimmune disease in childhood or in young adults. These cases are about 5 percent of all diabetics.

Yet both conditions are rapidly increasing worldwide. While considered separate diseases, they share an important similarity—in many cases patients use daily insulin injections to keep blood sugar stable. (Various oral medications may be used depending on the individual.)

My experience with diabetes began before entering private practice. I was diagnosed in the early 1970s. Fortunately, I knew enough about nutrition to immediately make the appropriate changes, which included better eating and physical activity. I am no longer considered diabetic, but could easily fall into that state simply by eating a typical American diet filled with refined carbohydrates—something I strictly avoid.

The Centers for Disease Control and Prevention (CDC) stays that, "Type 2 diabetes can be prevented through healthy food choices, physical activity, and weight loss. It can be controlled with these same activities."

In the coming years, the CDC estimates that a third of Americans will be diabetic. Today, the condition costs the U.S. upwards of a quarter trillion-dollars a year.

Diabetes appears later on the spectrum of carbohydrate intolerance. Abnormalities often begin early in life. Clues that health is impaired can even appear at birth. So we are often given plenty of warnings about potential future problems. Below are some common signs and symptoms of carbohydrate intolerance in adults and children.

In adults:

- Poor concentration or sleepiness after meals
- Increased intestinal gas or bloating after meals
- Frequently hungry
- Increasing abdominal fat, upper body, or facial fat
- Frequently fatigued or low energy
- Insomnia or sleep apnea
- Waist size increasing with age
- Fingers swollen/feeling "tight" after exercise
- Personal or family history: diabetes, kidney or gall stones, gout, high blood pressure, high cholesterol/low HDL, high triglycerides, heart disease, stroke breast cancer
- Low meat, fish, or egg intake
- Low fat diet
- Frequent cravings for sweets or caffeine
- Polycystic ovary (ovarian cysts) for women

People don't really die of diabetes—despite it being listed on death certificates—but rather from the harmful side effects of insulin. This includes heart disease, stroke, and even other chronic, preventable conditions such as Alzheimer's and cancer. So the game for all diabetics is to reduce reliance on insulin. Many are even able to eliminate it.

The same applies to pre-diabetics and others who are carbohydrate intolerant. These individuals produce too much insulin because of poor diet, and the goal is to reduce insulin production. The signs and symptoms listed above are examples of those directly related to the overproduction of insulin.

Long before diabetes is diagnosed, individuals on the carbohydrate intolerance spectrum, including pre-diabetes, produce too much insulin. The body can overproduce insulin for many years—as long as high glycemic carbohydrates are consumed. Included are cereal, bread, bagels, rice cakes, pasta, white potatoes, soda, sports drinks and bars, and, of course, sweets. (High protein diets can also cause too much insulin production.) These foods trigger higher levels of insulin resulting in some or many signs and symptoms.

This well recognized problem used to be called hyperinsulinemia—excess insulin. But that name was too cumbersome and didn't catch on. Today, the popular buzz phrase is Metabolic Syndrome. But unfortunately, it only names certain end result conditions within it, such as high body fat, high triglycerides and cholesterol (and low HDL), hypertension, and high blood sugar. It does not emphasize the cause—refined carbohydrates leading to excess insulin.

Why is there no longer talk of high insulin in those who are not (yet) diabetic? Or why don't health professionals strongly encourage their diabetic patients to significantly reduce, minimize, or attempt to eliminate their needs for insulin by eating well and exercise? Some do, but for most, it's easier to just give a pill, so to speak.

So who is the real villain here? The food industry certainly wants you to eat more junk food, which worsens all the problems highlighted in this section (and many others). Blood sugar control is also a huge revenue stream for the pharmaceutical industry. Both spend billions in advertising to convince the masses of their great products.

Insulin is hailed as a wonder drug, yet too much can be more harmful than heroin. The same can be true for the body's production of natural insulin.

Our insulin needs are lower than most think. The pancreas only makes more when carbohydrate foods are consumed, and in diabetics an increased dose of insulin is required. The problem can be seen even in a relatively healthy individual eating a typical American diet—insulin production may be twice that of a person consuming no refined carbohydrates. Reduce carbohydrate intake and insulin requirements can be greatly reduced.

Our muscles can actually obtain adequate amounts of sugar (glucose) without insulin. In fact, this occurs all the time during and immediately after exercise and physical activity, when insulin secretion is very low.

In addition, we are not dependent upon sugar for energy. We also can obtain significant amounts from fat, reducing reliance on sugar. Those who burn higher amounts of fat and less sugar are, overall, much healthier. But insulin impairs our ability to burn body fat for energy (the reason those exposed to higher insulin have elevated blood fats).

Of course, the most significant indication of one's vulnerability for diabetes, like the full spectrum of carbohydrate intolerance, is consuming junk food. Most is made up of refined carbohydrates— the many forms of sugar and processed flour. Healthy eating does not include any of these items.

Whether one is already diabetic, of either type, a pre-diabetic, or has risk factors for carbohydrate intolerance producing too much insulin, addressing the cause of the problem is simple—eliminate all refined carbohydrates. For some, further reducing natural carbohydrates can lower insulin production, or one's dose, even more.

Oversold on Sugar: Is the white stuff running you down and wearing you out?

Even if you think you're avoiding it you may not be. Sugar could be finding its way into the food you are eating. This happens during travel, in restaurants, buying packaged items, those holiday dinners, or if you don't make all your meals from real food. After more than a hundred years of sugar deception by the industry, three things have come into focus: a small number of companies have become huge conglomerates, regularly reaping billions of dollars in profit by selling sugar; second, billions of sugar consumers worldwide have become sick and fat, including young children; and the problem continues to worsen.

In discussing sugar, I include other processed carbohydrates too because they convert to sugar very quickly in the body after consumption. This includes flour and other refined carbohydrates found in breads, crackers, cereals, bagels, muffins, and other items, not to mention sweets—let's just call it all "sugar." It's impossible to say, but probably 99 percent of the sugar consumed is the refined, unhealthy version—the stuff that maims and kills. Unfortunately, for most Paleolithic people today it is a global food staple.

Governments have jumped on board the sugar bandwagon, long ago, encouraging citizens to eat more of these unhealthy foods. It's not just a problem in affluent societies. In the course of only one generation, many millions of Third World people have gone from starvation to obesity through the consumption of sugar. (The World Health Organization calls it the "nutrition transition.")

Clearly there are many health and fitness problems that result from the consumption of sugar. Here are some of them:

- Illnesses such as obesity, diabetes, cancer, Alzheimer's, stroke, high blood pressure, and heart disease.
- Chronic inflammation, a key part of injuries and other physical disabilities ranging from arthritis and bursitis to muscle, ligament, tendon and bone disorders—even hair loss.
- Fatigue and depression.
- Increased body fat.
- Poor oral health, including cavities, tooth loss, and gum problems.
- Lower quality of life—often part of the aging process, but the brains of young people are adversely affected by the regular consumption of sugar.

Abnormal sugar regulation can occur in those without diabetes or other diseases. Even in active people, including competitive and professional athletes, higher levels of body fat are becoming common. Despite expending a lot of calories in training, too many of these calories burned during a workout are in the form of sugar and not fat. This occurs because eating sugar effects metabolism, forcing the body to use much more glucose, and too little fat, for energy. The result is less energy for endurance performance.

Because less fat is used for energy, it's stored throughout the body in hopes it will be used someday.

Poor performance is often associated with sugar consumption. Whether you are a runner trying for a better race time, a golfer seeking lower scores, an executive or student wanting more brainpower, a pilot, machine operator, or commuter who cannot afford to make an error, reduced performance is associated with sugar consumption. (Probably many more auto accidents come from this than alcohol.)

The most common symptoms of excess sugar intake include sleepiness and loss of concentration, especially after meals. That's because blood sugar is reduced by insulin, depriving the brain of its constant need for glucose. Another complaint by those eating too much sugar is intestinal gas, often due to the inability of the body to effectively digest many kinds of sugar.

Sugar in Disguise

The myth of "whole grain" continues to lure millions of people into thinking they're eating well when, in fact, they are just consuming sugar. The same untruth is commonly told about sugar being necessary for energy. The fact is there is no nutritional requirement for sugar, including carbohydrates.

Agriculture scientists have made genetic changes to sweeten many of our natural foods, causing them to contain harmful sugar. These include potatoes, corn, watermelon, and pineapple. It is just as if you scooped up the white stuff with a spoon and ate it for dinner or a snack.

So even if you think you're not eating much sugar, think again: whether in a gas station store or Whole Foods, almost all bread, cereal, rolls, muffins, pasta, noodles, bagels, rice cakes, and foods made with refined flours are just sugar. Not to mention the junk food products with higher amounts of sugar such as cakes, cookies, candies, pies, and similar items sold in these same stores.

Of course, many liquid refreshments can cause even more harm because they are usually highly concentrated—especially colas and juice drinks. Likewise for so-called sports products (most are consumed by non-athletes), which are usually full of sugar. These include Gatorade and the many related beverages, carbohydrate replacement products, energy bars, and others. For athletes, just consuming these products during competition won't magically improve performance—instead, training the body to be a better fat-burner is the first step, then finding a healthy source of carbohydrate for competition can help maintain speed and endurance.

In addition to table sugar, called sucrose, many other names for different versions of the same harmful food are common. Here are some of them:

- Beet sugar
- Corn sugar, high-fructose corn syrup
- Rice syrup
- Maltose, malt sugar/syrup, maltodextrin
- Dextrose, glucose
- Fruit juice concentrate
- Grape sugar
- Invert sugar
- Molasses
- Raw sugar
- Cane sugar
- Sorghum syrup
- Turbinado sugar

If you read ingredient lists you'll find sugars listed everywhere; from ketchup and mayonnaise to cold cuts and fish products. There is even a separate listing for "sugar" under the "carbohydrate" heading on nutrition labels. Most, although not all, of these sugars are the added variety.

And don't be fooled into thinking that certified organic sugar is any better for you—it's not. This is just part of the deception.

Sugar is also hidden in many packaged, frozen, canned and otherwise processed food, sometimes not listed on the label. The ongoing name game with labeling is meant to deceive consumers, with food lobbyists petitioning governmental regulation so the products don't look so bad. It was not long ago, for example, that the only ingredient in peanut butter was listed as peanuts. But a sizable amount of sugar was added too. That particular loophole has been closed, but we usually only hear about these types of tricks after the fact, so beware of any packaged or prepared item. The same is true in most restaurants—fast foods are especially full of it, but most food services use sugar as a cooking ingredient.

If sugar, in any of its many forms, is a part of your diet—whether it is the majority or just smaller amounts—you will only be healthier and become more fit without it.

Another problem with sugar is that the bad foods containing it are taking the place of healthy items in our diet. Instead of fluffy, nutrient-poor unhealthy processed foods, replace them with the real thing, especially fresh fruits and vegetables, raw almonds and cashews, the best protein choices (including eggs, meats, and fish), and other foods as tolerated such as cheese and other fermented dairy, beans, and lentils.

If it would make the world a better place, why can't we just stop eating sugar? This is easier said than done for the millions of people who are hooked on the white stuff. There is even a so-called war on sugar in some local governments who want to keep sugar out of schools or reduce the amount of sugar in single serving items. It is certainly something to applaud. But like big tobacco, the sugar industry has a more powerful and secret weapon—addiction.

Many people encounter great difficulty giving up sugar in all its forms. Foods don't taste the same without sugar, they say. And because sugar is such a widely used ingredient, finding out which foods don't contain it can sometimes be a nutritional challenge.

Of all the patients I've treated for serious illness, all the fitness problems encountered in a wide variety of athletes, coach potatoes and everyone in between, the single recommendation that helped more people the most—probably more than all other therapies combined—has been the elimination of sugar. In fact, this seemingly simple, single recommendation can dramatically improve your health, reduce body fat, and increase performance literally overnight. Eliminate sugar today and you can be significantly better tomorrow.

Does this mean no more desserts or enjoyable food? Certainly not! While I avoid all processed food, I do eat a healthy, homemade dessert daily, sweetened with small amounts of natural honey or fruit. Honey is a lower glycemic food, tolerated well by healthy people and most of those transitioning from sugar addiction to a healthier lifestyle. My website contains a recipe section with many healthy desserts (see below).

It is our choice to be healthy or not, to perform well or poorly, to reach our human potential or continue to struggle, to be injured and in pain or to live life to the fullest—or, to finally shed the unwanted body fat.

Artificial sweeteners are a sham

I recommend avoiding artificial sweeteners in virtually all situations because I believe fake sugars can have an adverse effect on your health. Some say the research is still not clear on this issue, but I say why wait when there's enough information about its harmful effect? Their use is linked to various health problems from headaches to indigestion.

Artificial sweeteners are used in many food items: diet soda, chewing gum, ice cream, iced-tea mixes, and many other products. If you want to avoid them you must read the labels.

While substances such as saccharin are not recommended for children or pregnant women, and aspartame has been related to an increased incidence of migraine headaches and allergic reactions, another fact has been ignored: The use of artificial sweeteners is most often accompanied by increased consumption of food. In other words, if you use artificial sweeteners, studies show you often end up eating more food, usually sweets. What's worse is that you may store more fat as well. Researchers are unclear why this happens, but certain factors seem to be implicated. It may be a learned process by the body. The tasting of sweet substances may cause the body to store, rather than burn, fat. Or, it may be related to the dehydration that accompanies consumption of artificial sweeteners. This may trigger the brain to increase the appetite and food intake as a means of restoring water balance. Eating low-calorie substances will lower the body's metabolism. This will not only cause the body to store more fat but also activate the need to eat more food.

Some people argue that artificial sweeteners reduce calories. You may be fooled into believing that you are buying a more-healthful, low-calorie food when you choose a product made with fake sugar. But you're avoiding only 15 calories per teaspoon when using an artificial sweetener. This is not a significant caloric factor.

In recent years, alcohol sugars have become popular as a source of low calorie sugar. They include xylitol, mannitol, and sorbitol, with new ones being developed—but they all have a common feature, ending in the letters "ol." One of the newest alcohol sugars is erythritol—and it's certified organic!

They are a hydrogenated form of a carbohydrate. Xylitol is the most commonly used alcohol sugar, and is made from glucose. Alcohol sugars don't break down very well in our intestines and so don't get absorbed to stimulate insulin like regular sugar.

Beyond Fat Burning: The Ketone Body

Our body obtains energy from a spectrum of sources. These include sugar, fat, and ketone bodies, and even protein. The more energy we have, the more we can develop our aerobic system leading to better endurance performance.

Unfortunately, fatigue is still a very common complaint of many athletes. It is not normal to be tired, despite a lot of training. So if this is your case, it's possible to your overtraining, or you don't have energy, or both. (Of course, it's possible that other conditions exist, such as iron deficient anemia.)

Overall, those with lower amounts of energy are generally less healthy, have increased body fat stores, are injured more often, and don't move as fast, sleep as well, or age as gracefully.

Interestingly, despite fatigue being common, athletes still find ways to perform too many fatiguing workouts, many of which are anaerobic.

We obtain energy from food, but the makeup of every meal and snack dictates the value of that energy. In particular, how much we have, how long it lasts, and how much goes unused and stored in the body. We potentially can obtain twice the energy from eating fat than from carbohydrate and protein combined.

Consider these aspects of our metabolism:

- Up to half of the carbohydrates consumed are converted to fat and stored.
- When breaking down fats for high-energy fatty acids, glycerol is released and can be converted to a very small amount of sugar.
- Protein contains amino acids, some of which can be converted to sugar. This can be significant for those eating large amounts of protein.
- Our bodies also recycle other metabolic products—we reuse water, digest our own digestive juices and saliva (for additional protein), and we convert blood lactate into glucose, to name some interesting metabolic reactions.

Because both protein and fat can convert to sugar, our true need for carbohydrates is actually zero. Not so for protein and fat, which contain what nutritionists refer to as *essential* nutrients, meaning we must consume them to be healthy.

Very Low Carb Intake

As our intake of carbohydrate foods gets lower, more stored fat can be used for energy. With an even further reduction of carbohydrates more *ketones*—derivatives of fat—are produced and also used for energy.

Many people want more energy to train and race faster, achieve much better health, greatly improve brain function, and other benefits. This can be accomplished by going further up the energy spectrum. It involves reducing insulin more by eating much less carbohydrates so the body creates ketones from fats, a super high source of energy, which the brain and almost all the body can use in a healthy way.

The study I referenced at the beginning of this section ("Rethinking fat as a fuel for endurance exercise") discusses a condition called fat adaptation. Humans don't need to *become* fat adapted—we are already there. It's our normal, healthy physiological state. We just have to make sure it's switched on.

The mistake made over the past few hundred years (although the process began thousands of years ago) is that through misguidance and bad advice by governments and the food industry our bodies have been forced to be *sugar adapted*. This has not worked well, other than it has spawned a huge market for health care and pharmaceuticals to treat sugar-related illnesses. These include most chronic diseases, from Alzheimer's and cancer to diabetes and heart disease, not to mention the continually growing worldwide overfat epidemic.

While burning more body fat leads to better endurance performance, there are many other healthy features. These include increasing athletic longevity and preventing injuries to name just two. What more could endurance athletes ask for? The answer is burning even *more* fat.

The Ketone Body

Some people reduce carbohydrate intake significantly enough to produce many more ketones. Whether we call this fat- or keto-adapted, Paleo, or any number of other popular names, don't call it a "diet." It's a metabolic state.

When this occurs, our metabolism significantly increases the production of *ketone bodies*—a group of three natural chemicals produced in the liver from fats. They are also used for energy. (Technically, they are called *ketone bodies*, and not *ketones*.)

Ketosis is the metabolic state associated with a high amount of ketone bodies in the blood. It may be an important marker, a sign that you have reached a very high level of fat burning. This could bring virtually unlimited energy for longer and faster training and racing, and also speed recovery each day.

Just eating a high fat diet will not accomplish high fat burning or ketosis. Only a very low carbohydrate diet (and avoiding too much protein) reduces insulin levels sufficiently to allow maximum fat burning—breaking down more stored body fat and converting it to energy.

In addition to reducing carbohydrate foods, it is necessary to add more fats to each meal to make up for the reduction of calories from the significant reduction of carbohydrates. (This is usually easy because fatty foods are the most flavorful.)

Eating more dietary fat does not mean your overall caloric intake will be higher—often, in fact, it is the same. Sometimes, calories can be reduced as individuals who burn higher levels of fat may actually require *less* total calories. One nice side effect is that oxidative stress can be reduced—helping the immune system, controlling inflammation, and improving the pace of aging.

Measuring Ketone Bodies

The most popular way to determine whether your body is in a high state of fat burning and producing ketone bodies is through a simple dipstick test. Available in drug stores, this evaluates the presence of ketone bodies in urine. But it is only a general measure, albeit one that is adequate in most cases. To more accurately assess which ketone bodies are being produced, and in what volume, blood tests are most accurate.

More important is the fact that certain symptoms are associated with burning very high levels of fat and ketone bodies. With regular eating, one should rarely become hungry. So hunger is a common indication that fat burning is not sufficient. This is also true during training sessions. Those who require nutrients during long training are usually not burning adequate fat. Likewise for those requiring large amounts of carbohydrates during racing. Athletes who burn large amounts of fat for fuel can eliminate or greatly reduce nutrient intake during long events.

More Fitness Benefits From Fat

In addition to very high levels of fat burning increasing overall energy for the aerobic system to work better, there are other endurance benefits.

- Many athletes want to slim down, including achieving weight loss and reducing body fat. This can significantly lead to better economy, resulting in faster training and racing. Even a few pounds for an average sized person can make a significant improvement in an endurance event.
- The state of nutritional ketosis influences the body to use more fat for fueling muscles. In doing so, glycogen is conserved. This is important during competition, and for maintaining stable blood sugar during sleep.
- Increased fat and ketone burning also reduces the body's reliance on food and carbohydrate drinks *during* long training and competition. Again from "Rethinking fat as a fuel for endurance exercise," the authors state: "Common lore dictates consuming about 6000 kcal of carbohydrates during a competitive 100-mile race, but low-carbohydrate runners commonly finish (and often now win) these events on 1500 or less 'in-race' calories." Another example was highlighted earlier in this Section—Hal Walter

relied on water only during his five-hour world championship race.

- With more competitors rising in the age-group ranks, many also want to continue training and racing into their 60s, 70s and beyond without impairing performance. This can also be accomplished by burning high amounts of body fat. (This topic is discussed in detail in Section 9.)

More *Health* Benefits from Fat-Burning

Speedy Recovery

Because high fat burning and increased ketone bodies reduce inflammation and oxidative stress, we can recover faster from physical activity. This can even help us better tolerate the other stresses of life too. Without a healthy body, recovery takes longer because of increased production of free-radical stress. But with increased fat burning and more ketones, athletes could train better, race more often, and increase performance—the *trifecta* of endurance sports.

Inflammation and Free Radicals

The significant reduction in dietary carbohydrate also dramatically influences the body's balance of the inflammatory mechanism. The reason is simple: lower insulin reduces the production of inflammatory chemicals. This can reduce physical injuries, which are often associated with "itis" conditions such as tendonitis, plantar fasciitis, and arthritis, and problems elsewhere in the body such as gastritis, colitis, and others. Ketones also have a positive effect in controlling our genes, and in regulating free radicals to help speed recovery from a workout, a race, or a season.

The Brain

For about a hundred years, medicine has used a high fat-burning ketosis state to treat epilepsy in children and adults. This condition includes seizures, a serious sign of brain injury. Those who are successful can often reduce or eliminate the need for medication. However, since the development of antiepileptic drugs starting in 1930, these medications became the more convenient therapy despite "the continued failure of even newer drugs to offer significantly enhanced clinical efficacy" (*Jasper's Basic Mechanisms of the Epilepsies,* 2012).

The increased use of ketones and decreased reliance of glucose in the brain also provides other recognized benefits referred to as *neuroprotection.* From Alzheimer's disease and other cognitive dysfunction to Parkinson's, most brain problems are preventable. Protecting the brain is one way to accomplish this, and a healthy eating plan promoting high fat and ketosis can have great value. Other brain and head conditions that have responded well to ketosis include headache, traumatic brain injury, sleep disorders, cancer, autism, and multiple sclerosis.

Another important feature of eating well is a high-energy brain that's creative with great stamina, not to mention better learning and concentration.

Cardiovascular Disease

Lower carbohydrate intake can quickly and significantly reduce a variety of cardiovascular risk factors. Reductions in triglycerides occur rapidly in patients with high levels, typically within a few days. In addition, maintaining a reduction in carbohydrate intake can significantly balance cholesterol, lowering LDL and raising HDL, further reducing cardiovascular risk. Some individuals respond to modest amounts of carbohydrate reductions, while other must go further along the spectrum to ketosis for this to occur.

Low carbohydrate intake also quickly lowers insulin, which can significantly reduce abnormally high blood pressure. People should be cautioned that this sometimes happens in a few days, too. Those with hypertension who are performing the Two-Week Test or just going off carbs "cold turkey" should monitor their blood pressure carefully. A health professional can do this while adjusting or eliminating medication as blood pressure normalizes.

Carbohydrate Intolerance

Whether diabetes, insulin resistance, low blood sugar, or other names associated with the inability to properly metabolize glucose and insulin, these problems can change rapidly in response to healthy eating. By shifting metabolism to increase fat burning significant improvements in overall health follow. In fact, carbohydrate intolerance can diminish to the point where patients can live healthy lives often with reduced or no medications, including insulin. These changes can often take place very quickly too.

The Gut

By reducing carbohydrate intake, intestinal stress is often reduced, too. Starches and disaccharides can impair gut bacteria, not to mention cause a high amount of gas production.

Athletes who no longer need large amounts of carbohydrate during training and racing also get relief with significantly less gut stress. In addition, because of reduced free radical stress and lower levels of inflammation, those who consume less carbohydrate foods may have overall healthier intestinal tracts, often able to rid themselves of conditions such as colitis, gastritis, and other chronic gut disorders.

Hormone Balance

With increased fat burning comes better control of two important hormones, insulin and cortisol. Both can significantly influence other "downstream" hormones throughout the body. For both men and women, these include testosterone and the estrogens, important for regulating many body functions. While they are often reduced during periods of training stress and poor health, improving fat burning can help restore their levels naturally.

It should be noted that ketone bodies are continually being produced in the liver of a healthy body. There is no danger in raising these levels by reducing carbohydrates. But mention ketosis and some people think of a complication of diabetes—by not properly controlling blood sugar, ketone bodies rise to dangerous levels, reducing the blood pH leading to a serious condition called *ketoacidosis*. In a relatively healthy body, raising ketones is not only safe—it's normal and healthy.

With so many benefits of increased fat burning it would seem everyone would want to eat well. What may be the two most common reasons for people unable to maintain a healthy diet are sugar addiction and fat-phobia.

Our fat burning abilities are dictated by the macronutrient makeup of the diet. On one end of the spectrum, poor eating habits maintain our dependency on glucose for energy with a fat-storing, unhealthy metabolism. But by reducing carbohydrate foods we move along the spectrum to burn higher amounts of fat for energy, reduce body fat, and improve health. Moving *further* along the spectrum by lowering insulin even more, ketone bodies elevate considerably and contribute significantly to our energy needs, with additional fat burning raising endurance, and health, to even higher levels. Our place on the energy spectrum is all in our hands.

ECONOMY 101

"It's the economy, stupid." This cliché, which originated in Bill Clinton's successful 1992 presidential campaign, is still repeated in American politics today. I've used it myself, but in relation to a different kind of economy—that of the endurance athlete's body dashing down the road, spinning through the air, and whirling through water. In fact, body economy is directly related to race performance.

Consider the many factors that affect the competitive athletic body, from shoes and hydration to fuel and feeling pain. We tend to discuss each separately, even though we know the body is not a mass of separate pieces but one highly functional organized entity that's greater than the sum of its parts. That one factor that can sum up the workings of all the body's parts into a highly organized efficient system is economy, the hidden secret naturally contained within all of us.

A recent study by Wayland Tseh and colleagues published in the *Journal of Sports Science & Medicine* on the "Influence of Gait Manipulation on Running Economy" states that, "The magnitude of increases in VO2 reported in this study raises the intriguing possibility that meaningful improvements in running economy might be achieved by manipulating the gait of distance runners who exhibit specific aspects of running style that deviate markedly from the optimum."

This has been the foundation of my approach in working with athletes from the beginning. Physical imbalances can be corrected, and gaits can be improved. But that's only part of it—improving the dietary intake, building the aerobic system, and others discussed here are important factors that can improve health, balance the body, and lead to a better gait with improved economy.

Body Economy

Each day, millions of endurance athletes go out to train and, invariably, sometimes subconsciously, images of the great runners, cyclists, swimmers, and other near perfect-looking athletes are in our brains. While the greatest athletes seem to expend relatively small amounts of energy to coordinate legs, hips, shoulders, and arms to drive their bodies to great feats, when we go out to try the same the outcome is usually not the same—we can't go as fast or look as invincible. That's because for most of us, our bodies are less efficient, or economical, than those few picture-perfect bodies so frequently portrayed by the media and in movies.

In fact, we expend *more* energy covering the same distance, and just as hard, but get less in return. The reason for this is well understood—certain physical, chemical, and mental-emotional factors can interfere with the brain's ability to move the body with the same efficiency as a great athlete.

What distinguishes the best endurance athletes from all others is *body economy*. It is not a theory, nor psychology, but our natural physiology. It is not genetic, luck, or some special skill gifted at birth. All endurance athletes have the ability to run, bike, ski, row, or swim with higher levels of efficiency, giving us grace, and more speed.

Improving body economy is the single most important factor that can dramatically improve your sport. But economical improvement is not a single act, like wearing special shoes, or an emotional mantra that helps us focus in a race. Instead, it is a composite of all our physical, chemical, and mental factors that funnel through the brain and into the body, allowing effective and highly efficient movements, helping to unlock the natural power of the body's abilities.

One way to accomplish this task is *not* to think of these great athletes. Instead, it's important to focus on our own bodies, allowing the brain to do what it does best: organize the most efficient movements.

The *potential* for great economy is what we all have in common with the greatest endurance athletes. While most may never get to that level of athleticism because too many roadblocks are in the way, each step we take toward it means more efficiency and a better race.

So the goal is to improve body economy by removing the roadblocks that prevent our brains from making the body do what it already knows how to do. First, we must recognize these barriers and then reduce their negative impact on the body, or eliminate them altogether.

There are many specific ways to improve economy. They include making the muscles more efficient, and to do that the brain must work well too, since it controls all movement. The feet must function optimally since they are the foundation of all body actions. Energy in the form of fat and sugar must be generated and properly balanced so we can endure two, four, ten, or more hours of competition with sufficient energy to maintain those great movements.

Imagine the brain as a big funnel, and through it goes all the various physical, chemical, and mental activities that influence your movements. When these factors are working well and funneled through the brain into the body, improved economy results, along with better training and improved racing.

But if we funnel *imbalances* through our brain, the body won't work nearly as well. The barriers to improving body economy are many. They include muscle imbalances, reduced foot function, poor fat burning, a less-than-optimal heart, lungs, and circulatory system, and other physical, chemical, and mental factors.

The human body is made to be athletic, evolving for millions of years into a great movement machine. Body economy is a priority for the brain, which naturally wants the body to be both highly efficient and effective in all movements. This is not limited to endurance sports, but also daily chores, working on the computer, and even rolling over in bed. We all posses the ability to move well, with accuracy and without wasted energy. We just have to remove the roadblocks.

Often without realizing it, athletes actually try to improve body economy in at least one of three ways: through training, understanding the body, with nutrition, and various self-help methods—not to mention a little help from their friends. But despite the focus on some of the activities that can help improve endurance, often with great intensity, and as it should, greater body economy often eludes them.

This is because improving only some factors that can help body economy without enough of the others won't get the body beyond a certain threshold in improvements—the reason many athletes improve to a point, then plateau. As important as having the right mental state, a high VO_{2max}, the best equipment may be, if muscle balance is not adequate, or energy waning, to note just two such examples, body economy will only progress so far but still be less than optimal.

Body economy is expressed best in a balanced body and brain. No matter how hard or detailed you try to compete, movement won't be optimal unless there is good balance in an adequate number of key body parts. These include muscles, bones, hormones, and nerves, to name a few. The bottom line: You decide how much you want to improve by choosing how many roadblocks to remove so economy improves past a certain threshold—one where you're suddenly performing your best at any age.

An individual's economy is not static. It can change from one week to the next, or over the course of a season or lifetime depending on wear and tear, recovery, and overall health. All along the way it will parallel an individual's performance. That's because the brain is always changing—working better on certain days compared to others. This is another important feature of great economy—consistency. Having a relatively high level of economy more of the time separates the better athletes from the rest. So just how do we improve our body's economy? Most of what I write and lecture about are factors that can significantly accomplish this task. When working with athletes one-on-one, it's the focus of my attention, where it's easier to fine tune someone's body for improved economy. Below is a review of some of these factors.

Factors That Make You Faster

For endurance athletes, most of the talk about improving performance revolves around VO_{2max} and lactate threshold. Despite their popularity these two factors are more important for relatively short, middle distance events, like a 5K, than for marathons, triathlons, or ultra events. The trendy measurements can be misleading. VO_{2max} does not predict longer performance outcomes, which most people race around 85 percent of the VO_{2max}, such as for a marathon, to 70 percent typical of an Ironman performance. These efforts are very close to, or under, max aerobic training. (During these endurance races, blood lactate levels are closer to resting levels than a 5- or 10K race.)

Getting faster is most easily accomplished with better movement economy. Often related to oxygen utilization, improving economy simply means training to run, bike, or swim faster at the same heart rate. When training with a sub-max heart rate, I recommend the 180 Formula. And you'll know when body economy is improving—you'll go faster at the same heart rate. Here are some practical and useful ways to accomplish it. The first two important factors have already been discussed: building a great aerobic system, and increased fat burning—the important combination of training and diet. Other include:

- **The Feet.** As we know, the energy to train and race from comes from both sugar (glucose) and fat. But through a unique energy return system in our feet (and lower legs), we have the ability to harness the gravitational impact forces from hitting the ground, turning it into additional energy. This extra energy can be significant. But it won't work well in feet that are dysfunctional. Muscle imbalance, overstretched tendons, inflexibility, and other problems render many feet unable to obtain this extra energy. Spending more time barefoot, even just walking around your home or office, could be the start of an important rehabilitation process that allows better foot function. If you are already doing this, venture out more, performing some barefoot runs and walks. The result can be improved running economy.
- **Running Shoes.** The main cause of poor foot function is bad shoes, especially when running. These are the ones that are not a near-perfect fit. In addition, those that are too heavy, over-supported, thick soled, with a higher heel can impair foot function too—this means most training shoes and racing flats. Wearing any shoe for training and racing will reduce running economy. The goal, if you must wear shoes, in addition to improving foot function, is to minimize the problem by finding the ideal shoe for your foot.
- **Muscle Balance.** Even a slight irregularity in one's gait can reduce running economy. Muscle imbalance is usually the cause of gait problems, causing the body to expend more energy than necessary. It may be associated with an injury or overtraining, both of which impair normal muscle balance. Correcting the cause of this problem, which may be due to footwear, diet, training, stress, or other factors—and often combinations—will allow you to get faster at the same sub-max heart rate. Pain itself can disturb

muscle balance. Whether due to poor joint movement, inflammation, or other reasons, pain usually means you're doing, or have done, something wrong in training. Finding and fixing the cause of pain should be a priority.

There are two important ways to correct muscle imbalances. First, be as healthy as you can. In this situation, the body fixes many of its own problems, including muscles that don't contract properly. Second is the potential need to find a healthcare professional who can perform therapies that correct muscle imbalance. This may also involve improving muscle strength. A surprising number of endurance athletes have poor muscle strength, especially those past age thirty.

- *Food.* The foods we eat can directly affect running economy by improving fat burning, balancing muscles, increasing circulation, controlling free radicals, and helping to build a better aerobic body.

- *The Brain.* It's the most misunderstood and most neglected part of an athlete, yet, it's the most important by far as all the above factors are regulated by it. It's the brain that improves the body's movement economy when the roadblocks that prevent it are removed. The brain takes your slower workouts and is able to make you faster. This has to do with practice performance, allowing your body to go through the proper motions at a slower pace allowing the brain to do it faster with more economy.

- *The mental-emotional state.* Interference in economy can be the result of misinformation, usually from bad advice. The images we see on TV, of lead runners in the marathon traveling sub-five-minute paces, remain in the brains of millions of athletes who jog along at a ten-minute pace in the same race. We all want to run that way, but we can't. And we should not pretend, either. Another mental-emotional factor is bad posture. Remember what your mother said, or your teacher: "Don't slouch—sit up straight!" It's easy in our society to develop bad postural habits.

We devote a lot of energy to some movements, like running or lifting weights, but neglect other activities like healthy posture. The result is that we slump at our desks, stand with poor posture, and even walk with a bad gait—all because somewhere along the way we allowed our bodies to get lazy. For many, these bad habits carry over to running.

Enhancing these factors discussed here in my Big books, even by modest amounts, can significantly improve body movements such as swimming, biking, and running economy. The result will be training and racing faster at the same heart rate.

Live High, Train Low

If you are very serious about improving economy, here's another factor: Altitude.

For decades, endurance athletes have sought altitude training as a way to get faster. But this is misleading. *Living* at higher elevations, such as seven to eight thousand feet, can help develop the aerobic system and improve running economy. The ideal situation is as follows:

- Living at higher altitude, 7,000 to 8,000 feet.
- Training at lower elevations, 4,000 feet or lower.
- Racing at lower altitude can improve race times.

But just going to altitude does not guarantee results. That's because the process requires a healthy body. A poor diet, for example, may not supply all the nutritional needs, such as iron, folic acid, or protein, necessary for altitude living to increase quality red blood cells and better aerobic function.

When Gait Goes Bad

Why are many endurance athletes significantly slower than others? Of course, there are as many answers as there are runners, cyclists, and others who train and race throughout the world on a regular basis. But an important general answer is that it's due to an altered gait, which reduces economy. Simply looking at most top finishers of a marathon or Ironman, and comparing them to those mid- or back-of-the-pack, and we can easily see what a poor gait looks like. In this section I will discuss a variety of factors that can worsen gait and lead to poor economy of movement.

Body language is millions of years old, and has played an integral role in helping humans survive as a species. Our sitting and standing stance is called posture, and the way we move, regardless of the activity, is referred to as gait—these are the words of body language.

In a natural setting, the brain "reads" another person's body language thanks to cells called mirror neurons. (All animals use it to identify weaker prey, a potential healthy mate, or an enemy to avoid.)

Our stature, body language, or gait is a reflection of the body's physical, chemical, and mental-emotional state, and is the sum total of our health and fitness. This complex mechanism is regulated by the brain, which controls the individual muscles that move us, producing our particular gait.

We move in specific ways, at particular paces with varying qualities. A vibrant youthful gait is significantly different from one that is less balanced, bent over a bit, or limping. Even a seemingly insignificant injury, a minor metabolic problem, or a bad meeting with the boss can adversely affect whole body movement through the actions of muscles.

When our gait goes bad, we slow down, whether we are washing dishes, walking to the market, or running a marathon.

For decades, researchers have been studying various aspects of the human gait. Sports scientists watch athletes move, neurologists measure patients with brain disorders, and various clinicians—from chiropractors and medical doctors to massage and physical therapists—assess muscles when performing a comprehensive evaluation.

This information can help piece together the cause of an irregular gait, and the potential injuries or illness that may be related.

More serious conditions can make themselves evident through an altered gait even before other signs or symptoms arise, making this evaluation an important tool for predicting impairments. Here are some common and easy-to-see examples of measurable altered gaits slowing people down:

- A limp is typically due to some foot, lower limb, or back injury.
- Patients with neurological impairments usually have an obvious irregular gait, including those with Parkinson's, multiple sclerosis, stroke, and other brain injuries.
- Illness such as vascular diseases affects gait too, including those who had a heart attack.
- People with impaired memory, from those without obvious signs or symptoms to patients with more severe cognitive dysfunction such as Alzheimer's in its earliest stage, show gait alterations.

The evaluation of gait has obvious value in sports. Observing an athlete's actions can provide important clues that certain muscles may not be working well, increasing the risk of injury. But even if that injury never occurs, the resulting irregular gait will still slow the pace, whether walking, running, cycling, swimming, or any athletic movement. By correcting the cause of the abnormal gait, injuries can be prevented and improved performance restored.

With an irregular gait, the muscles are working ineffectively, and the body's energy is being used less than optimally. It takes more effort to go from point A to point B with an irregular gait, which also elevates the heart rate more than usual, making one fatigue faster. And, it increases physical stress on joints, tendons, ligaments, and bones. The brain, which monitors all these activities as part of its body protection plan, slows our movements rather than risk further damage to an already fragile frame.

The Economy of Tempo

Humans move at paces with incredibly similar fashion regarding cadence or tempo, despite differences in our natural gaits. Most of us run about 180 steps per minute. A healthy individual normally walks at a basic pace of about 120 steps per minute. Even our daily activities have been shown to have a "pace" of 120 steps or moves per minute. One exception is walking or running on a treadmill, which is unnatural—the brain senses the body's movement but remains in one place. The result is a wider variation in tempo.

Another exception is when the gait is significantly altered, which not only slows us down but also reduces our ability to maintain a healthy tempo.

These numbers—180 and 120—are not precise but an average. Virtually all runners have a *range* of tempo between about 150 and 190 steps a minute whether jogging, running a marathon, or sprinting. This allows the brain some leeway to adjust one's pace and gait as necessary. Muscle imbalance, fatigue, caffeine, time of day, the weather, and even the estimated time necessary to complete a workout or race can all influence one's gait. The brain will sense these factors and make appropriate changes such as slightly slowing our tempo, or speeding it up, and increasing or decreasing stride length.

Improving one's gait starts with finding the cause or causes for it to be altered—especially the individual muscles that may be contributing and the reasons for their imbalance. Muscle dysfunction in the foot is a frequent cause of altered gait. But nutritional factors, poorly fitting shoes, mental stress, and other features of our overall wellness can contribute too. Just improving health can help one's gait, sometimes significantly. This is the best recommendation for getting gait—and performance—to a better level.

Fitness affects gait too. Poor aerobic metabolism, for example, can reduce muscle endurance. In addition to its contribution to fatigue, related to more reliance on sugar for energy and less on fat, this problem can also influence gait.

Music can help the brain improve the gait. In a recent study, Dr. Andrea Trombetti and colleagues of University Hospitals and Faculty of Medicine of Geneva, Switzerland, demonstrated that listening to music increased the brain's ability to better balance the body. Music stimulates the brain's rhythm centers in the cerebellum, which strongly effect physical activities controlling gait. But I don't recommend listening to music *during* a workout. It's best to listen to your body. Instead, I encourage athletes to play music whenever possible, especially during down times, as a way to relax, and during meals (which can help digestion).

Stretching Can Disturb Gait

In evaluating muscle function in athletes, one factor is outstanding—stretching a muscle could make it longer, and this can result in a reduction in function from a loss of power. Stretching can cause *abnormal inhibition*—weakness. There was a consensus on this issue by many, although certainly not all, clinicians. By stretching muscles before running, it's very possible to cause muscle imbalance with the result of irregular gait.

Muscle damage from stretching will obviously have an adverse effect on an athlete's gait. The loss of smooth efficient movement puts stress on virtually all other structures—ligaments, tendons, joints and bones, in addition to many muscles. The body tries to compensate for this irregular movement, and in doing so uses up more energy, taking away from one's performance. A recent study by Jacob Wilson and colleagues at Florida State University showed how stretching can result in poor running economy, increasing energy consumption during an endurance event, and decreasing performance.

Carefully conducted human studies have shown that stretching decreases a muscle's force production capacity, causing weakness.

These side effects of stretching are demonstrated in various ways by measuring muscle function using electromyographic, dynamometer, mechanomyographic, and similar devices commonly used in human research. One particular study, conducted by J Cramer and colleagues from the Department of Kinesiology at the University of Texas, compared changes in muscles that were stretched and not stretched in the same person. It concluded that, stretching one muscle can also impair another one that's not stretched, possibly through a central nervous system inhibitory mechanism. In other words, by weakening a muscle through stretching, the brain and spinal cord may trigger other muscles that are not stretched to become weak, as well. This occurs even in muscles in the opposite leg.

While the studies show that these abnormal changes induced in a stretched muscle can last for an hour, some clinicians have demonstrated that stretching can cause prolonged muscle problems that can last days and weeks.

Gait Pain

Pain is an emotion. It can wake us up at night, can keeps us off our feet by day, and otherwise create a significant stress for our body and brain. The result can be time off from training, impaired race performance, and significantly reduced economy.

Pain originates in nerve endings (pain receptors called nociceptors) found in the skin, blood vessels, nerve fibers, joints, and coverings of bone. These pain receptors send messages to the part of the brain responsible for emotions (called the limbic system), where we interpret the feeling as pain.

Acute pain is typically the result of some kind of trauma—a cycling accident, a twisted ankle on a trail, or just bumping our knee, hand, or head into something hard. This pain lasts a short time while the body is healing the damage done. In this case, the cause of the pain is well understood.

However, sometimes pain appears in a muscle, joint, or, more often, somewhere more vague and difficult to pinpoint. The pain sometimes builds up from a seemingly dull ache to a more serious discomfort. Inflammation often becomes part of the pain syndrome. The developing chronic pain may cause the body to compensate by making different movements—the brain literally changes our gait to reduce movement or gravity stress on a certain joint or muscle.

This chronic pain may be due to at least three possible problems.

- First, the problem that caused the pain is unresolved. For example, a muscle imbalance causing stress in the knee joint can cause inflammation and pain. Until the cause of the problem is corrected, both inflammation and pain continues.

- Second, in some cases, even when the physical cause of the problem is corrected, chronic inflammation is maintained. This is a chemical imbalance associated with poor fat balance. Until this problem is corrected, pain chemicals (including those causing inflammation) can continually be produced.

- There's a third possibility for persistent pain even when the physical and chemical causes are resolved. Certain types of brain cells, called glia, the most common ones in the brain, can become overactive following some injuries or imbalance. These cells continue to stimulate the pain even after the original cause of pain has resolved. What triggers the glia to become overactive is not well understood, but certain pain medications, especially morphine, seem to actually worsen this process. Other substances can potentially turn off the overactive glia. These include cannabinoids, the active component in marijuana, as can stronger prescription drugs (immune suppressant drugs such as etanercept, and narcotic receptor blockers such as naloxone).

For most athletes, pain comes from the musculoskeletal system, and develops from muscle imbalance and altered gait. Often the dysfunctional movement is painful by itself prompting athletes to seek medical help or attempt to remedy the problem through self-therapies that might include cryotherapy (cold), natural remedies (such as anti-inflammatory foods or dietary supplements), or over-the-counter or other medication. (The various aspects of pain, drugs that affect it, and their many serious side effects, and natural ways to control or eliminate it are discussed in detail in the *Big Book of Endurance Training and Racing.*)

In this situation, clear causes are difficult to diagnose even with modern technologies (X-ray, MRI, and other imaging techniques) because the problem is a functional one. Clearly defined structural damage has not yet occurred. This is the condition most athletes encounter.

If the body is unable to correct the problem, whether with assistance of a therapist or self-remedies, the altered gait can continue stressing the body and over time pave the way to pathological changes in muscles or joints. These are also seen in athletes, especially those with a history of acute injury (a fall), metabolic disturbances that contribute to a stress fracture, or other more serious causes.

How does the brain adjust the gait to avoid some imbalance, no matter how subtle? A runner may shift weight to the inner foot as it hits the ground, which could lead to secondary ankle and foot injuries. Swinging the arms too much could cause misalignment in the spine. And many other adaptations can occur in cyclists, swimmers, skiers, and in any other athlete with the result of an even worsening gait leading to poor economy.

In addition to poor-fitting shoes, improper bike set up, or other equipment, spending too much time sitting in the course of the day can also have adverse effects on gait.

Sitting Stress Can Ruin Gait

We all sit at times. But minimizing it can help improve body economy. The stress caused by more than short sitting time is not just associated with physical problems, from back and hip pain, to neck and headaches, but increases the risk of disease.

For millions of years, the human body squatted rather than sat. It was the normal posture, one compatible with overall health. Squatting not only helped muscles, bones, joints and other structures function well, but helped other areas too, including the body's circulation and intestinal function.

Over the last few thousand years, humans made a bad move by sitting more and squatting less. Of course, in some cultures, squatting is still popular today. And all young children can comfortably squat. Most of the world's great endurance athletes can squat well, while most others are unable to accomplish this simple biomechanical task.

Perhaps the most unnatural physical position for the human body is sitting in modern chairs and seats, whether in your car, office, airplane, or at the dining room table. For all people, including athletes, prolonged sitting is associated with significantly more injuries, ill health, and even disease, all leading to an earlier death, compared to those who sit much less.

This information is not new—scientists and clinicians have been studying this public health hazard for decades. The most recent research comes from Hidde van der Ploeg and colleagues at the University of Sydney. Their study of 222,497 men and women forty-five years and older, published in the *Archives of Internal Medicine* (March 2012) showed that those who sat the most—eleven or more hours a day—are 40 percent more likely to die within three years than those who sit less.

The average adult spends 90 percent of their leisure time sitting down. This involves eating, socializing, and, most especially, watching TV. While those in the study who were physically active had fewer effects from sitting stress, those who were inactive and sat the most had double the risk of dying within three years.

Sure, it's relaxing to plop down in a La-Z-Boy and take it easy after getting home. How harmful can that be? The fact is, our modern society offers seating opportunities everywhere. Our early ancestors never had these so-called luxuries—for millions of years they squatted and stood almost all their waking hours, and rarely sat like we do today. So our bodies have not adapted to today's unnatural sitting position. Seats are so plentiful that most people spend more sitting time than they realize, devoting much of their day to doing it.

The technology trend in chair ergonomics over the past few decades was supposed to rescue us from sitting-down stress. The technology claims to cure aching backs, necks, and shoulders. But it hasn't, despite the commercial success of businesses specializing in "body-contour" office chairs, car seats, toilets, and even back rests. While comfort is the most important factor in determining the best chair for work and leisure, and the most appropriate car seat position, sitting is almost a no-win situation. The less you sit the better.

Sitting's Double-Edged Sword

Sitting stress is a modifiable life-style behavior. Generally speaking, it can result in two separate patterns affecting our health.

- One is associated with more metabolic problems. This means more body fat, higher blood pressure, blood sugar problems, even cancer, heart disease, and diabetes. This is the mechanism that can lead to an early death in those who sit the most. For many years, scientists have been studying those who spend more time sitting, demonstrating that various aspects of our metabolism can become impaired. The reasons include reduced muscular activity, especially of the lower extremities, with associated decreases in blood flow, and can literally deform blood vessels. There is also a general stress stimulus that could contribute to reduced health just like any physical, chemical, or mental stress impairs body function.

- The second pattern affects our biomechanics. This may induce muscle imbalance, tendon and ligament impairment, and joint stress. It's the reason increased sitting can cause, contribute to, or maintain a physical injury. The unnatural positions of sitting in modern chairs, car seats, and couches place the pelvis in a stressful position causing the whole spine to twist, flex, and extend in order to compensate for this unnatural position. In turn, this affects the shoulders and arms, and thighs and legs. In particular, your joints are most affected, from those in the pelvis and entire spine, to the hips, shoulders, and even the jaw joints. Muscles take much of the brunt of sitting stress, which is not unlike wearing bad shoes. To keep the body from getting too twisted, the muscles try their best to compensate for such unnatural positions—some get tighter while others weaker. This, in turn, has a bad effect on your posture and gait. Once the muscles start making these changes, literally sacrificing their normal activity to prevent joint, bone, or ligament damage, you get used to sitting without feeling bad.

I'm not talking about avoiding all sitting, but for those who spend a significant amount of time sitting down—which is the majority of people, whether active or not—reduce the time spent in that unnatural position as much as possible. This means being on your feet more instead of hitting the couch or chair. It also might mean creating a standing workstation, which involves having your computer, writing surface or other items higher up off the desk so you can stand and work comfortably, such as positioning your computer at a higher level that's easy on your arms, hands, head, and eyes.

It does take a little more energy to stand compared to sitting. This occurs because you use more muscles. And until you get used to this posture—a couple of weeks in most cases—you may not be able to take the jump from a lot of sitting to much more standing overnight.

Reclining, even just using a footrest, sitting on the floor, and even lying are more natural positions for the body. But the goal should be more standing and less sitting.

> With additional standing you'll not only remain more mechanically stable with better muscle function, as the months pass you'll burn significantly more calories to reduce extra body fat.
>
> Of course, there's a catch: To really reap the benefits of less sitting you have to be in reasonably good aerobic shape, and only wear good or no shoes. You just might be amazed how much better you feel.

Finding *Your* Perfect Gait

It's important to understand that there's no perfect athletic form everyone should follow. While all humans have the same *basic* patters of movement—just like other animals—our individual styles are ours alone. In fact, it's easy to recognize your running partner from a distance, even before the face comes into focus, because you know his or her unique running fingerprint, their gait. (I will talk about the *running* gait because it's easier to identify, but cyclists, swimmer, skiers, and all other athletes have unique body movements we can also call gait.)

Look at athletes in all sports and there's one common feature—everyone's movements are slightly different.

However, if something interferes with our natural movement—something that causes our gait to go astray—two things can happen.

- First, we may get injured. An injury means something went wrong, and while it may be caused by a poor gait, the injury will in turn worsen the gait more. All this will be reflected in running form in a very subtle, or sometimes in a more obvious way. Irregular movement in the hip joint, more flexion of the knee on one side than the other, too much rotation of the leg, and erratic arm movements are some examples. The most common reason for this is muscle imbalance, forcing the body to compensate by contracting certain muscles more to keep the imbalance from worsening. All these actions lead to poor economy.

- The second problem is that we are unable to effectively train with a high level of efficiency, and don't compete up to our potential. No matter how painful or hidden muscle imbalance is, it reduces economy. This can be seen during a daily workout—trying to run at our race pace will raise the heart rate more than usual, making us fatigue quicker and slowing down sooner. This is how the MAF Test can give a clue that some mechanical imbalance has developed, impairing gait and economy.

Adapting to Habits

Humans adapt well to the environment, often very quickly. The brain adjusts to the weather, our physical bodies, and race terrain by metabolizing and moving differently to seek an optimal pace. We adapt to both the good and the bad. Here's an extreme example. Let's say you weigh 170 pounds. Place a fifty-pound pack on your back and start your normal run, and within a few steps you'll adapt to the stress. Now you're running with a different gait, and more than likely, it's the appropriate one for your body when carrying a fifty-pound backpack. The brain senses the added weight, assesses the body's ability to compensate, sends messages to certain muscles to contract harder while others relax more, and thousands of other directions are given and within a half dozen steps you are running, albeit with a different gait that your brain decides is acceptable. This won't be a pretty gait, but it will be as effective as possible considering the circumstances. Obviously, it will slow you down, as well.

Another common bad habit occurs when you put on a pair of running shoes that don't match your feet, and therefore the rest of the body. Maybe they're too small, too narrow, or just too thick. Whatever the problem, your body adapts to the shoes as best it can. In doing so, the mechanics of the whole body can become altered.

Whether you only have one bad habit or have accumulated many, in order to run with a natural economical gait, you have to retrain your body. I should say that your brain has to retrain your body. Otherwise, you may never find that optimal running form.

The Best Running Gait

In the *Star Wars* movie classic, *Return of the Jedi*, Obi-Wan Kenobi makes the now famous statement, "feel the force." If you want to move properly, effectively, faster and without injury, one key factor is your ability to feel the force. But if you are talking throughout your workout, listening to music or just not paying attention to your body, it may not happen.

What force is that? Gravity. Instead of it working against you, as is the case when gait goes bad, make it work in your favor—improve it.

I'm often asked about the best way to run. What's the best running form? As if there is a checklist everyone should follow. Fast turnover? Lean forward? Push off?

I wish it were that easy.

What *is* easy, however, is the notion that if your feet hit the ground properly, the rest of body tends to follow with a gait more naturally tailored to fit your body. While this is the most important place to start improving your gait—and if there's a problem here's the one to fix first. But this is easier done than said.

Many sports shoes interfere with the feet doing their job, which could cause the whole body to have a poor gait, inducing stress into muscle, bones, and joints. A specific problem that's most common is that many running shoes cause you to land on your heel instead of further forward on your foot. Over time, this causes, among other things, muscle and other problems in the feet. Now your body's foundation is cracking at the seams.

Feet Affect Gait

The fastest way to feel your ideal gait is to take off your shoes and run barefoot—at least for 50 or 100 meters. By eliminating interference between your feet and ground, you may quickly have the best form. Among other things, this will improve your foot strike—from heel to forefoot—produce better pelvic movement and arm swing, and allow your head to better control eye and body coordination (a very complex but important part of running efficiency).

By doing this, you should feel a different gait right away. I don't recommend everyone become a barefoot runner, although it might improve many body imbalances, and race times.

One of the missing parts to most of the discussions about barefoot running is the fact that just walking around without shoes—not running unshod (without shoes)—but just weight bearing with naked feet, is exceptionally therapeutic. This simple action can ultimately fix many feet.

Think about getting a great foot massage. That's what your feet feel when you're barefoot. They get to be free, they move without restriction, and the muscles ultimately work better. Potentially, it's their favorite way to move—at least if they have not already been damaged. In this case, being barefoot may not feel so great.

Feet that don't function right are a problem for both the feet and the rest of the body too. Your feet are your foundation, your contact with the ground, and a vital source of energy during a run (the arch mechanisms work in such a way that its spring-like motion takes a lot of that pounding force and recycles it for use as energy).

Perhaps the most common problem that athletes develop in the feet is muscle imbalance. One way to correct it is to find a healthcare professional who can figure out which muscles are not functioning and fix them. Another way to fix your feet is to stimulate them in such a way so as to enlist the help of the brain, and all the muscles, ligaments, tendons, and even the skin. We all have our optimal running form programmed into us from early years of development; from our brain to all the muscles, the information is there. Being barefoot helps our body return to our best form, as many of us had in our youth. It may be one of the key reasons that East Africans continue to be the best endurance runners in the world—they spent their lives developing their brains and bodies barefoot.

As adults, it's not necessary to train or race barefoot, but just to spend time at home or work without shoes. Walk on the grass barefoot, even for ten minutes a day. The more time barefoot, the more your feet will work better in a shoe. But the shoe must fit well, be flat and not interfere with your normal foot mechanics. This will help with proper landing, which should be on your mid- or fore-foot during running. Once your feet are happy, you have the best chance at better running form. The feet are discussed in more detail in Section 4.

Good Gait Habits

Do we need to create textbook marathon runners who look like they're racing eight hundred meters? Can we really take each component of gait and make it picture perfect so we can run faster with the same or less energy? The answer to both is no. Instead, just run in a comfortable, upright position. It could be that simple. However, there's a problem if we've trained ourselves to lean forward too much, or we try to stride like a world-class marathoner, or have learned other bad postural habits that interfere with our natural gait—we need to break them. Here are five common factors that can help you break some stubborn habits.

1. Avoid the "Perfect" Gait
You can't fool Mother Nature, so don't mess with gait. Instead, do the most you can to remove the roadblocks that prevent you from producing the best form your brain can create in the body, such as wearing proper shoes, not mimicking other athletes, and overall, being healthy (which corrects many of the body's physical imbalances).

2. Don't Lean Forward
It seems obvious. If you lean forward you'll fall forward, so it must be a good way to run. It's not. The problem with *leaning* forward is

that it's too often accomplished by *bending* forward. This is not only unnatural, but a stress on the body. This added stress results in an altered gait, the use of more energy, and an impaired economy.

Instead of bending at your waist, or tilting forward, which flexes the pelvis, think about the whole pelvis being slightly more forward. Properly done, this will allow you to run in a more upright posture. Think about being taller when you run, which technically you are. As the spine becomes straighter (now that you're not slumping forward) you will also want to make sure your head is in a natural position too. Do this with your eyes and your head will follow: look slightly below the horizon—not gazing straight ahead, not looking up, not with your head dropped down hoping to move your body with the weight of your head forward.

By bending or tilting forward, the stress causes the powerful *gluteus maximus* muscles in the area of your butt to weaken because they now contract less (which causes the quadriceps on the front of the thigh and possibly the psoas muscles in the front of the pelvis to tighten too much). And, both the lumbar (low back) and cervical (neck) spine extends too much, producing an exaggerated curve along with extensor muscle tightness in the back of the neck and low back. It's not a pretty picture.

All this makes the body use more energy to accomplish the task. This could also cause weakness in the neck flexor muscles in the front of the neck, making the head less stable, which can further worsen your form. When running, think about a forward pelvis and you'll feel your quadriceps contract as you hit the ground with your foot. If you do this correctly, you'll feel your butt tighten, and even produce slight muscle soreness between workouts due to chronic *maximus* weakness—they get sore because now they are working well for the first time in a while.

This may be difficult to do if you wear over-supported or thick-soled running shoes because you'll land on your heel, which forces your pelvis to be back instead of forward. By wearing proper shoes and landing mid- or forefoot, your gait is more likely to be optimal. Landing hard on your heels will never allow the body to have a great gait.

Pushing off is not something you need to consciously do each step. Your brain will take care of that action. Pushing off should be natural and occur without you doing anything if your gait is right. If we have to force our push-off, we're probably doing something wrong, such as wearing the wrong shoes. In that case, the pounding becomes a negative and ultimately can contribute to an injury.

3. Fast Turnover?

A fast turnover is fine, but can you just run faster and disregard your brain and body wanting to slow you down? Can you mimic that great runner with the eight hundred-meter type long stride while in a marathon? No. Just like you can't shorten your stride too much to get a faster turnover just because, well, faster must be better; that could be a significant stress on your gait as well. If too long or too short a stride is unnatural and stressful, what's left is the ideal stride length for your body—an important part of your own personal gait. If you wear a heart monitor, you'll see that over- and under-striding both raise the heart rate. And finding your most relaxed gait will produce the lowest heart rate. The result is you'll train, and race, faster.

You can run within your own natural biomechanics and without overtraining to accommodate a faster turnover as if in a race by performing *downhill workouts*. By running down a moderate grade (not too steep) you can maintain the same heart rate and run at a much faster pace, thereby having a faster turnover. This was discussed in Section 1.

4. Tempo

Humans move in incredibly similar fashion regarding tempo. All our runs are "tempo" runs; likewise for biking, walking, hiking, swimming, and skating. As endurance runners, we all run about

180 steps per minute. We all walk at a basic pace of about 120 steps per minute. Even our daily activity has been shown to have a "pace" of 120 steps or moves per minute.

The exception is on a treadmill, which poses a particular stress due to its unnatural circumstance—the brain senses the body movement but the body remains in one place. In this case there's a much wider variation in tempo.

These numbers—180 and 120—are approximate and are an average. Virtually all runners have a range of tempo between about 170 and 190 steps a minute. This allows the brain a bit of room to adjust our pace as necessary. Muscle imbalance, fatigue, caffeine, time of day, the weather, and other factors can affect our running economy for a given workout, and the brain will sense these factors and make appropriate changes such as slightly slowing our tempo, or speeding it up.

It's more than the brain, the rest of our head is important too, not only influencing tempo but gait. Our eyes (a part of our brain) play a role, as does our inner ear, which contains a tiny "otolith" on each side. These contribute to collecting information about body movement and balance. In addition, various muscles around our neck and those of the jaw joint (which connect directly to the brain as opposed to all other muscles which first connect to the spinal cord) continually send messages to the brain about body movement, and help the eyes and ears do their work. All this feedback in the head, combined with that from the feet, spine, pelvis, and elsewhere, helps the brain better adapt to many necessary moment to moment changes during our run. Most are subtle and not even noticeable. The result is the most efficient run possible. In order to do this, the brain may decide 176 is a good tempo, at least for the first twenty or so minutes, then it may change to 182, and so on.

5. GOT RHYTHM?

It so happens that humans have a rhythmic brain, and the walking tempo of 120, and 180 for running, are examples of our natural built-in neurology—the brain and nervous system—in all we do. Ask anyone to tap out a rhythm with his or her fingers and the tempo will usually be around 120 beats a minute. Even listening to music at this tempo is preferable. Scientists have evaluated more than 74,000 pieces of modern music between 1960 and 1990, and found that the average rhythm was around 120 beats per minute.

It is no wonder music can help our running, like all other sports, but not *during* a workout. At all other times, music can promote the activity of the cerebellum, that "little brain" at the base of our brain, which controls tempo and rhythm. People who can't maintain a smooth gait while running may benefit from listening to music—not in the background, but focused music as therapy.

How do we run faster? For most runners, this occurs with a slightly longer stride, with only a minimal increase in stride frequency. These changes are within the limits of your optimal gait—usually within the 170 and 190 steps per minute range.

My recommendation is to not try counting your steps during a run, especially avoid trying to run at a 180 steps-per-minute tempo as this could consciously disrupt what your brain is trying to subconsciously do.

Before trying this out at home, or I should say, on the road, understand the concepts. With the exception of being barefoot, which, in a few strides will immediately give you the idea, conceptualizing is as important as implementing. After all, you may have developed bad habits by learning the *wrong* concepts about gait. Just looking at a video of a some of the great-looking marathon champions, especially if someone says, "here's how you should run," does two harmful things: First, it instills that picture in your brain. Now going out for a run means thinking about that picture, even though you can't break seven-minute pace in a 5K. Second, just looking at the video, and each time you think of it during your run, the brain tries to imitate that world-class gait. While this may work for certain basic human movements, such as when learning swimming or cycling technique, running is more natural and we already have it built into us—the bad habits just overshadow it. So conceptualizing the good habits described here (there may be others based on your particular needs) is a great place to start creating your own personal perfect gait.

Of course, there's nothing like seeing to better believe how your gait really looks. To do this, there is gait analysis.

Gait Analysis

Endurance activities such as running, biking, skiing, swimming, and others that evoke consistent movements are associated with obvious gait images. Viewing an athlete running around a smooth track, for example, especially when watching from various distances with different views of the athlete from the front, back, and sides enables us to observe slight irregularities. In addition to stride length of each step, the changing cadence, body lean, side-to-side movements, foot plant and other specific actions, a trained professional can see more. An example is the runner who toes out on one foot. This may be caused by a particular muscle problem, sometimes more than one. In some cases, an abnormal function of the psoas muscle can produce this type of gait imbalance. In particular, a so-called "weakness" of the psoas allows the limb to rotate outward producing the toe-out gait. A professional who can evaluate the psoas muscle may also be able to quickly correct the problem.

This example may be the only problem seen in one runner, or it may be one of many other muscle imbalances disrupting the whole body. This latter example is often the case in those with significant gait irregularities, making observation, and determining which imbalances are most primary, a more difficult task.

Attempting to self-remedy of this problem may actually further complicate the picture. If a runner recognizes the unilateral toeing out problem, for example, and tries to compensate by rotating the leg inward while running, this can worsen the gait over time (sometimes immediately) because the *cause* of the imbalance is not addressed. The brain is already compensating for the problem, and trying to consciously alter the gait may override that process. Treating a secondary symptom is obviously something to be avoided because, in this example, it can lead to other muscles become over-worked or positioned in a way to cause further damage. (This is assuming that our runner has a primary problem with the psoas muscle.)

This is also the reason to avoid trying to make yourself look like that 2:04 marathoner when you can only run that distance in three hours. So don't try this at home!

Types of Gait Analysis

The above example is one way to observe someone's gait and follow up with additional assessments leading to a specific therapy. In fact, this has been a significant part of my personal approach when working with athletes. In today's high tech world, the process now includes computerized evaluation of a runner on a treadmill, bike, or other situation specific for one's sport.

There are many ways to evaluate a moving athlete. The full range of gait analysis goes from simple observation, which many coaches the health professionals have done with great success over the course of many decades, to very complex computerized dissection of each body part performed in a laboratory.

Many untrained individuals are happy to offer opinions about your gait, which might include a running partner, spouse, or even a stranger. Coaches and trainers often observe an athlete's gait, and sports stores sometimes have some type of evaluation that might include visual inspection of running shoes or treadmill assessment.

Sometimes a more specialized analysis is performed on a treadmill or other device and is often videotaped, allowing slow-motion inspection of certain movements.

Various kinds of sports practitioners and researchers frequently employ the use of more sophisticated studies such as digital video analysis with computer software that can produce two- or three-dimensional images. All the numerous methods provide different information. Accurate interpretation is what makes any one method much better, and one of the most important factors in being an expert is experience in performing gait analyses.

Despite the popularity of sophisticated gait analysis, regardless of the type of evaluation—from simple to high tech, the most important component is what comes next.

Any gait analysis resulting in some suspected abnormal finding should lead to further assessment that helps specify what type of therapy, if any, is needed. This might include a physical evaluation leading to the treatment of muscle imbalance, a recommendation of certain types of shoes that best match the foot, maintaining a good posture without slumping, or training at a more precise heart rate. Therapy should be directed at correcting the cause of a problem discovered by analyzing the gait and not just consciously changing your running form (which can be valuable but must be done with caution).

Just as important is the re-evaluation. If a problem is discovered and a therapy rendered, feeling better is an important indication of success. Even more important is the ability to run faster, for example, at the same heart rate. Re-testing using the same methods is vital to ensure that a problem previously observed no longer exists.

Measuring body economy as a way to demonstrate improvement is an important option for athletes. While this is traditionally accomplished by measuring oxygen utilization, it can most conveniently be done as an MAF Test discussed earlier and reviewed in Appendix B.

If you want to race faster, quicker training paces at the same heart rate are essential. Being a healthy athlete free of physical imbalances can help make this possible. This implies improved economy—the bottom line for better endurance.

OUR FEET,
OUR FOUNDATION

Proper mechanics involve harmony of all of the body's parts. With rare exception, such as when swimming, the foot serves as the link between some surface such as the ground or pedal, and the rest of the body. Without a secure, highly functioning foot, power can be lost during training and racing, and mechanical instability maintained or created leading to injury and lost economy.

The foot is such an important and amazing part of our anatomy that its importance in endurance sports could easily fill many volumes, and is the reason I've been writing about it for the past three-plus decades. The foot's many functions include maintaining position and balance and leverage for propulsion, and providing the foundation for all structures of the body above. During the gait movements, foot motion facilitates compensatory actions of muscles and joints throughout the body, particularly in the lower extremities.

While the feet influence virtually all structures above, up to, and including the head, improper alignment throughout the body potentially, in turn, can also affect foot function.

Let's start by discussing one of the important aspects of foot function, the nervous system and the relationships between brain and foot.

Is Your K-Sense OK?

Optimal movement starts with good foot-sense.

You're familiar with the senses of smell, taste, and sight; foot-sense is not as well known but is equally important. Imagine stepping out of the shower and your foot lands on a tiny pebble. The body reacts immediately by contracting certain muscles throughout the body, with the end result of lifting the foot off the ground. Likewise, a swollen joint in your toe is easily noticed with weight bearing on it; a tiny splinter seems innocuous except for each time you take a step on that foot.

The brain has reserved more neurological representation for the feet than most other areas of the body (the others include the hands, head, and neck). This is accomplished by the many nerve endings in the feet that communicate with the brain.

Foot-sense is the result of millions of nerve endings at work throughout the feet. They're found in muscles, ligaments, joints, and in the skin, and they sense tension, movement, force, pressure, and even temperature. Except for the spinal cord, there is more nerve activity in the foot than anywhere else in the body.

If you study the structure and function of the foot, such as in an anatomy-and-physiology class, you would learn the word for foot-sense is *proprioception*.

Among many other things, foot sense (or proprioception) allows us to determine the best pair of shoes that match our feet when we first put them on. Which are the most comfortable is the question answered by foot sense felt on a conscious level in the brain.

Just as important, the foot senses details about ground contact with each step, the effect of pedaling on a bike, or skiing in a boot. In doing so, the foot plays a major role in regulating all body function.

Through sensory information, you can successfully remove your foot from a painful pebble, adjust your cadence, or alter your gait as necessary to help compensate for some irregularity. In effect, you orient your whole body during standing, walking, running, and all other weight-bearing activities as a result of foot sense.

But the feet don't stand alone. All the nerve endings there sense and send important information—about the foot's movement, tension, pressure—up through the spinal cord to the brain. In turn, this allows the brain to influence the whole body in response to foot sense. This body-wide activity is called kinesthetic or k-sense.

Because of k-sense, you don't have to look down to see the position of your foot when standing up because your brain already senses its location. The same is true with the sense of movement—one doesn't have to look at each and every footstep, or watch every arm and leg movement in order to walk or run effectively. The brain already knows what's going on thanks to sensations from the feet (along with other senses throughout the body as well). Every step we take relies on k-sense.

K-sense can also be observed while balancing on one foot. The brain interprets incoming messages from the foot one is balancing on and sends back messages to muscles throughout the body to continuously adjust the posture to keep from falling. These movements may include tilting the head, moving the arms up and down, or whatever is necessary to keep balanced.

Imbalanced muscles, overuse injuries, disease, and infection can cause poor foot-sense, leading to distorted k-sense and increased vulnerability to further injury, poor posture, and irregular gait. The result could be lost economy—physical activity requires significantly more energy, slowing you down.

Many types of ill-fitting running shoes, including those that are oversupported and too thick, can also put stress on the foot's delicate structures, including muscles, bones, ligaments, joints, and even the skin. In addition, shoes that have a difference in height between the front of the foot and the heel can be a stresser—the natural foot on the ground has the same height front and back, but a shoe with a thicker heel causes the front of the foot to drop further down.

These problems can contribute to a local injury in the foot, such as blisters, bruising, or a first metatarsal inflammation due to the front of the toe jamming into the shoe or boot during movement. This, in turn, can further interfere with foot sense, further worsening communication between foot and brain producing poor body-wide k-sense. (Conditions such as diabetes, heart disease, and other illnesses that impair circulation are associated with deterioration of the tiny nerves in the feet rendering them even more dysfunctional. This leads to poor foot-brain communication and can significantly impair balance even when walking on a smooth surface.)

One result of poor k-sense could be that the brain is less aware of the body's foot precise position, with overall body posture altered leading to mechanical stress. The result is a response from the brain to the muscles throughout the body that may not be correct. As such, the body may not properly compensate for a minor foot problem, or even the normal wear and tear of training. This, ultimately, can lead to an injury such as Achilles tendonitis, or problems in locations other than the foot, such as knee or hip pain, or worsening of an existing problem like low back dysfunction.

K-sense Therapy

Who doesn't like to have their feet rubbed? Even babies love it. (I have only occasionally seen some patients with such significant foot problems who didn't want their feet touched—adding any stimulation further intensified insult to an already altered foot.)

You can use foot sense and k-sense to your advantage as therapy. Because the nerves in the feet dramatically effect foot muscles and balance, and communicate with the brain, stimulating them during normal foot movement can excite foot sense. This can be extremely helpful for the whole body, even when performed for relatively short periods. This is a key benefit of being barefoot—the most natural of all positions for the foot. It not only improves foot sense but can also produce full body benefits by improving k-sense. The results can be better muscle balance, improved posture, and more efficient gait. And, of course, this can improve economy.

Barefoot therapy can be done with almost anyone of any age, even for only 10 minutes per day. So just walk around the house, yard, or neighborhood to experience the benefits of going unshod.

Most athletes also spend considerable time in shoes they don't wear during training. These shoes must also fit perfect. However, the more time you spend on your feet after taking off your shoes, the more therapeutic actions you receive.

Injury-sense

A common reason for many foot injuries is poor foot sense, and improper k-sense. This may be the result of longtime wearing of shoes with thick shock absorbing material that make up the sole. The thicker the tread, the harder it is for the brain and foot to properly communicate with the body. In other words, the soles of the feet can't stay in touch with the ground. Sure, the over-developed shoe bottom is striking the ground, but there's a lack of foot sense not allowing for optimal body wide k-sense.

The relationship between reduced foot sense, poor k-sense, and its contribution to injury has been understood in scientific circles for almost forty years.

It's easy to see that trail running requires good k-sense. The uneven surface requires a significant amount of back-and-forth activity between foot and brain. In fact, this terrain can be a healthy addition to training on smooth roads, producing a healthier foot to help avoid injury.

But everyday activity can also be an obstacle course for one's feet. If you're walking through a crowded restaurant dining room to get to your table, you may have to squeeze past chairs, people, other tables, and perhaps even navigate your way across a wet, slippery floor. You rely on our natural k-sense to do this, and the process begins with good foot sense. Those who have worn thick-soled sports or casual shoes for enough years will have significantly reduced foot sense, and therefore k-sense, and will need to look down and around to keep from colliding into a chair, table, or person. But with properly functioning k-sense, you won't have this problem.

Testing Your Proprioception

The powers of proprioception can be disturbed by the slightest anomaly such as an abrupt uneven stretch of street, a protruding stone on a trail, or sudden unexpected change from a hard to soft surface. The end result can be a stumble or even a fall.

One day New York City filmmaker Dean Peterson set up his camera at Brooklyn's 36th Street subway stop. There on a staircase, one of the steps was slightly higher than the others, but by only a half-inch. Yet that seemingly insignificant difference caused many to stumble while ascending the stairs (subway stairway design guidelines call for risers to be a minimum of six inches and a maximum of seven inches). The mischief-making step has since been repaired, and you can view the video here: vimeo.com/44807536

Here is an example of proprioceptive deception you can do at home: Walk up and then down a flight of stairs. Can you tell there's a difference between the heights of the different steps? The communication between your foot and brain may be fooled, or even impaired, resulting in not knowing when a slight deviation occurs in walking stairs. In the case of the New York City stairway, it's a relatively minor increase in the height of one step.

Stair steps are supposed to be very similar in height, with local building codes dictating specific measurements. Many locales mandate, for example, that the difference between steps should not exceed three-eighths of an inch. That's because climbing stairs, and descending them, can raise the risk of falls when a height discrepancy is too great. The half-inch higher step in the video is clearly too much for many people, especially after having just walked up a number of stairs that don't have such a deviation.

We have taught our brains, through past experiences of climbing stairs, to expect each step to be almost the same. So when one is a half-inch higher than the previous ones, exceeding the brain's expectation, you stumble.

Ascending stairs is different than hiking up a rugged trail with a similar incline but lots of obstacles. When ascending a footpath, your brain expects each step to be a uniquely different height, and it helps the body compensate in at least two ways. One is through visual senses, which involves looking at where you're walking. A certain deviation, between one step and the next, if large enough, would be seen. The minor deviation on the subway staircase was probably not visually noticeable.

Another way the brain compensates is through information received from each foot as it makes contact with the ground. It does this all the time when we're on our feet. Nerve endings, especially those in your toes and the bottoms of the feet, immediately sense the ground with each step, sending very specific details of what it feels—hardness and softness, levelness, slippery or secure, and the like—to specific parts of the brain. This information reaches an area called the cerebellum in the back of the head and the mid-brain. These locations evaluate what the feet have felt, an assessment is made regarding balance and the risk of falling, and this information is then sent to the motor cortex—in the top-middle of the brain. Here it's decided which muscles throughout the body to contract and move for the most appropriate body response to the odd step.

All this occurs in much less than one second. The outcome can be easily seen in the video: when people begin to stumble on the higher step, with seemingly erratic, but really well organized movements of flailing arms, bending backs, and tilting heads, they quickly "catch" themselves thereby preventing a fall to the ground. Those with better foot-brain function have minimal hesitation, while those with ineffective function stumble more.

No doubt, the camera caught some individuals who did not have any problem with the higher step, and these were edited out. Or, the numbers of people in New York with poor functioning feet are very high (most of those in the video appeared to be wearing bad shoes). Those with better communication between foot and brain also appeared to be more fit individuals, who would have quicker reaction times. In addition, those who walk these stairs every day, probably most of those in the video, should train their brains, often sub-consciously, to adapt to the impending danger. But for this to happen, the foot-brain connect would have to be working well.

Back to your experiment: In your bare feet, walk up and down your stairs and using only your foot-brain sensation try to feel which steps are higher or lower than others. Carpet, like thick and soft supported shoes, will distort your ability to do this. If your feet are not healthy, it will be impossible to feel the height differences. (Of course, there may not be any significant changes from one step to the other, but like the subway steps, many builders and inspectors are not as careful as they should be). Once you think you feel any changes in height, get a ruler and measure the steps to see how well your feet and brain are aware of these subtle differences.

One of the Greatest Feats: 1:59

What will it take an athlete to run a sub-two hour marathon? That's easy—great feet.

I believe if the East African endurance athletes maintained their barefoot running habits, instead of getting shoe contracts and wearing racing flats, we would have long ago seen a sub-two-hour marathon. Kenyan Dennis Kimetto is one I previously deemed in my recent book, *1:59*, to have this potential.

With his day-glo orange racing flats flashing through the Berlin streets, Kimetto blazed to a world record 2:02:57 marathon in the 2014 event. The weather did not hinder his pace, and it may not have helped much either, as other race times were not particularly quick (third-place men's time was almost 2:06, and the women's race was won in more than 2:20). This made Kimetto's victory more him and less Mother Nature. The traditionally fast flat course in Berlin frequently sets up great race times. But on this day, the world record was only one of the important features of his day.

The morning after the great race finds many more runners, including those in the media, coaches, and sports scientists, not just talking sub-two hours, but believing in it. Beyond the fact that Kimetto's time was a world record, other factors helped fuel the 1:59 bandwagon—which, from this point on, will gain speed and build like a blazing runner in their final kick before breaking the tape.

Only recently have media questions started being seriously asked about a sub two-hour marathon. Such was the case in Berlin. Post-race, both Kimetto, and runner up Emmanuel Mutai, who also ran under the now old world record, were asked about it. The two fastest marathoners in history were clear and confident: "I am expecting a marathon in two hours," said Kimetto. Mutai agreed, claiming, "Today showed that the time is coming down and down. To beat two hours is possible."

In my analysis of the world's top marathoners, there seemed to be only a few today who appeared most likely to go under two-hours. That analysis was based on various factors such as fitness, health, and age. Along with Kimetto, Geoffrey Mutai and Wilson Kipsang (as I only found out after my analysis happen to all be training partners) are in the lead pack of potential candidates. (No doubt others are closing in, including non-East Africans from around the globe.)

The talk of the running world was that Kimetto's new record was a surprise. Not to Dennis, however, whose pre-race comments about his fitness level heading into the event were very positive. The proof was in his performance, and he took a great leap forward in his quest for 1:59. And it appears he's bringing much more of the running world with him.

The reasons for my choice in this great marathoner were many, and included his relatively short running career (only since 2010), one that is steadily improving. He is relatively young at age 30, and appears to have not yet peaked as an endurance athlete. Kimetto could have almost 10 years to continue improving, if he stays both healthy while building more fitness. Just as important, he believes a 1:59 marathon is real.

Two hours, three minutes and some odd seconds has been the marathon record for a seeming long time. The official marathon record has been "stuck" in various versions of 2:03+ since this same twenty-eighth day of September in 2008 when Haile Gebrselassie dug under the 2:04 barrier on the identical Berlin course. This year was Kimetto's turn to break through the next ceiling, into the 2:02 arena.

But this race resulted in more than the rapid rise in sub two-hour speculation—it gave an important sports psychology-type edge that marathon times will not only continue improving but just may do so with a more rapid acceleration than the improvements in recent years, which have only crept along. After all, a quick look at marathon record history shows that records are sometimes broken with larger leaps.

In the coming months, as another new record falls, look for a silencing of most of the emotional critics who claim that breaking two hours for 26.2 miles is impossible in our lifetimes. (Very similar beliefs were popular before Roger Bannister's sub-four minute mile race.)

Athletic achievements like Kimetto's always come with grand celebration and quiet retrospective analysis. Questions like, what went well with training, and with the race itself? And, what could be improved for an even better performance the next time around? This is where things get really exciting.

Even before the celebrations wind down, Kimetto and his "team," including his manager, coach, and family would have started planning for the next world record, with a continuation of the ultimate goal a bit down the road—1:59 and change.

In order to accomplish these tasks sooner rather than later, we must look at certain physiological factors—specifically, problems that can interfere with acquiring faster race paces. As great as Kimetto's world record performance was, in hindsight we see that certain adjustments in training and racing could have made his world record time quicker, even with the same effort. How much faster, of course, no one knows. Addressing these issues can obviously not only help Kimetto but also the handful of others jump closer to what will be considered perhaps the greatest of athletic feats, the 1:59 marathon. Below are some of them.

Steady State

First, consider the difference between running a marathon at a very steady pace, and one that is inconsistent, with faster and slower mile splits. It's like driving our car for two-plus hours, constantly speeding up and breaking to slow down—this would result in using much more gas (energy). While running, consistency in pace improves economy too. In other words, maintaining very similar (even close to identical) mile spits on a very flat course—what I call a "smooth" race—the body can cover 26.2 miles faster with the same effort. This did not happen in Berlin. Mile splits were slower than record pace early on, and even at the 15K mark leaders were about 30 seconds slower. Then, things got faster. Soon after the 15 kilometers Kimetto and Mutai ran a very fast 5K in 14:10. These patterns of speeding up and slowing down—faster and slower than one's average pace, creates poor economy and slower finish time. How much slower cannot be accurately calculated, but it is possible that Kimetto could have run 45 seconds faster at the same effort had he maintain the same miles splits on the flat course.

Part of the problem with accomplishing pace consistency has to do with a relatively new tradition for humans—wearing shoes.

Barefoot and Fast

Being barefoot is a way of life in East Africa, but also a choice many athletes make throughout the world. I've spent most of my life barefoot, even if I don't include sleep times. Growing up without shoes may be one of the reasons Kenyans and Ethiopians have dominated middle and long distance running since the Sixties.

Those brightly colored racing flats that Kimetto wore were more than shiny new shoes. They are an important part of a precise strategic marketing plan on the part of a large business conglomerate seeking to sell more shoes to both athletes and non-athletes. Wearing shoes is also how Kimetto makes a living. However, he might be better off financially if he ran without them. Why?

Kimetto, along with the very few who are capable of ultimately breaking two hours, built their bodies by being barefoot throughout childhood—the period when the brain and body developed muscles and fluid movements. It is one of the reasons their gaits are so seemingly near perfect. However, by wearing shoes, the return energy system naturally endowed in all our feet and lower legs may not work quite as well. The result is that an athlete uses more energy to race at the same pace, which ultimately reduces race times. Harvard's Dr. Dan Lieberman's research shows that running barefoot may be a full 5 percent more economical than wearing shoes. For more than a few great runners, the barefoot factor alone may be sufficient enough to go under two hours.

By running barefoot, something Dennis could probably quickly be race-ready for next time out, we could not only see another world record—perhaps in the 2:01 arena—but it would make everyone, including non-athletes, aware of the countdown to 1:59.

Emmanuel Mutai finished in second place in Berlin (and also bettered the old record). To keep pace with Kimetto he should not try training harder, but smarter. Immanuel may be a frontrunner in the second pack of elite marathoners with the potential for 1:59. Like all endurance athletes who want to not just survive but also thrive well into their thirties (Meb Keflezighi won the 2014 Boston Marathon close to his 39th birthday), overtraining must be avoided at all costs.

Be Both Fit and Healthy

At various points in their careers, too many of the world's greatest athletes are affected by significant injuries. This not only impairs progress, but also limits competitive years. All elites know their time is limited, so every day counts. Avoiding injury is a key for the crop of great runners seeking 1:59. A running injury is not normal, and it is preventable (barring unforeseen trauma such as a twisted ankle on a trail run). An injury means something went wrong—in training, or with other lifestyle factors that influence the body (such as diet and stress).

After working with athletes for almost forty years, I think it's clear that overtraining may be the greatest enemy. It can wreck the body, and end a career prematurely. Associated with overtraining is poor health. Like injuries, this can also adversely affect running economy—preventing a marathoner from reaching his or her true potential.

Don't Follow the Money

Runners must follow their own career paths. But keeping an eye on the big picture is almost a requirement for success. Nothing should interfere with training and racing. By most economical standards, top professional athletes make a great living. But if the business of running interferes with training and racing, causing fitness and health issues, world records often don't come as easy. The reason is that athletes, like everyone else, can become too distracted—literally causing excess stress—in the course of running their business (and despite having others around to manage their affairs). In addition to the relatively small contracts being offered to runners (particularly compared to athletes in many other sports), including those from shoe companies, they are quite small compared to the huge financial potential the first 1:59 runner could encounter—a real pot of gold at the end of the rainbow.

Consider that runners must promote themselves—their "brand." This means getting their face in the media with a lot of TV, radio, and print interviews. Business, promotional, and other appearances grow in number, including those scheduled right up to race day. No doubt this is already happening to Dennis Kimetto more than he has ever experienced. Potential sponsors are circling around him, asking for endorsements and offering contracts.

Marathon history, like in most sports, shows that world records will continue to be run, despite the epidemic of less than optimal training, poor race strategies, running in shoes, excess stress, and other factors that can reduce economy and slow the rate of new records, with the next one right around the corner. It's just a matter of time. When it comes to the 1:59 marathon, the question is who wants to step up and accomplish this inevitable feat first.

Some sport scientists predict marathon times of under two hours, and even well below that level—even sub 1:50s (which also means women will ultimately run 1:59). The only question now is when it will happen. While no one knows the answer, it is clear to increasing numbers of people that it can happen in the coming few years. Even more important is that a small handful of elite runners believe it most strongly. The countdown to 1:59 continues.

The Earliest Foot Problems

Children's shoes may be a primary cause of physical problems later in life. That's because footwear can impair normal neuromuscular development.

In those athletes with foot problems, most come from shoes. But often, the sports shoes, boots, and even casual wear just worsen existing problems. Where do these foot problems originate? Typically in childhood.

More than twenty years ago, a review of shoes and gait in the prestigious medical journal *Pediatrics* outlined some key factors that affect children's feet. Pediatric orthopedist Dr. Lynn Staheli, from the Children's Hospital and Medical Center, Seattle, Washington, listed these important points:

- Optimum foot development occurs in the barefoot environment.
- Stiff and compressive footwear may cause deformity, weakness, and loss of mobility.
- The term "corrective shoes" is a misnomer.

- Shoe selection for children should be based on the barefoot model.
- Physicians should avoid and discourage the commercialization and "media" obsession with faddish footwear.
- Merchandising of the "corrective shoe" is harmful to the child, expensive for the family, and a discredit to the medical profession.

Perhaps the most offensive aspect of the footwear industry is the harm it deliberately inflicts upon unsuspecting children by encouraging them to wear bad shoes. Between the twin forces of television and parental encouragement, little Johnny or Jill are defenseless. In particular, the potential damage to the young developing body and brain. And this could be a primary cause of physical imbalances, injury, and disability later as adults.

It was evident from Dr. Staheli's article that shoe companies in 1991 were already heavily marketing unhealthy children's shoes, playing on the parent's emotions and those of older children. Today, shoe companies continue to use clever million-dollar advertising campaigns to encourage kids to ask for, and parents to buy, harmful shoes.

And it's obviously successful. The U.S. children's footwear industry, which includes shoes for kids up to sixteen years of age, generates more than $5 billion annually, where products are made for cuteness and style rather that sacrifice function.

What's the best shoe for your child? None—barefoot is best and nothing comes close. Children should be barefoot most of the time. This provides the optimal stimulation of the foot by the ground, which helps train the brain for proper gait and other natural movements that children require from the start. Unimpeded, a healthy barefoot child's gait is essentially perfect.

When a shoe becomes absolutely necessary, Dr. Staheli says it should be lightweight, flexible, shaped more or less quadrangularly, and should not have arch supports and stiff sides. She says that pediatric orthopedists strongly oppose "corrective" or "orthopedic" shoes for straightening foot and leg deformities like flat feet, pigeon toes, knock-knees, or bowlegs, claiming there's no evidence that these so-called therapeutic shoes are effective. Instead most of the supposed deformities in children naturally correct themselves. How, you might ask?

Being barefoot is the best way for that to happen. Most health-care professionals who properly understand a child's body mechanics know this. (Yet there are many "experts" who recommend the regular use of shoes for young children, but they are usually aligned with the shoe industry or companies making orthotics and other corrective devices.)

Any shoe has the potential to seriously disturb the gait of a young child. His or her sensitive feet sense footwear much more than the adult foot. Even relatively minor pressure on a child's foot from a shoe can begin deforming it, leading to a permanent problem.

During the first year following the acquisition of independent walking, most of the child's gait activity, in particular, the neuro-logical memories—the communication between brain and body—becomes well established. During this time, if the feet are not allowed to develop well, gait and balance disorders begin to occur. In many children, these irregularities are often subtle (the "clumsy kid") while others more serious such as increased vulnerability to physical injury and various neurological imbalances anywhere in the body, including those associated with eye movement.

The full development of a child's balance and compensatory mechanisms, and overall gait mechanics, takes years to mature. While the first five years of life are most delicate, neuromuscular interference from footwear can occur at any and every stage along the way into early adulthood. This can lead to more serious and chronic physical imbalances later in life, such as a running injury or back pain, and even amplify the stress caused by imperfect shoes.

Earlier this year, Caleb Wegener, PhD, and colleagues from the University of Sydney, Australia, reviewed the problems associated with a variety of different shoes worn by children for walking and running. Their study, published in the *Journal of Foot and Ankle Research*, states that, "Shoes affect the gait of children. With shoes, children walk faster by taking longer steps with greater ankle and knee motion and increased tibialis anterior activity. Shoes reduce foot motion and increase the support phases of the gait cycle. During running, shoes reduce swing phase leg speed, attenuate some shock and encourage a rearfoot strike pattern." In short, these are some of the specific items that are a recipe for physical and neurological disaster, and the start of a process of chronic injury and disability that could last a lifetime.

These researchers noted Dr. Staheli's twenty-year-old suggestion that shoe design should be based on the barefoot model. But some of the shoes they tested were designed on these principles and still caused gait irregularities in children.

The researchers also state that, "Further attention could also be paid to reducing the weight of shoes which may be responsible for some of the [abnormal] changes found in children's walking and running gait." (It's interested that this type of "free" information is available to shoe manufacturers but may never be utilized—instead, they test their shoes on machines, not real people.)

Among the untold problems that wearing shoes can impose in the developing child is the impact on the brain. From a baby's very first delicate steps, each walking and running gait pattern significantly influences brain development. These actions affect lifelong patterns in the nervous system, even beyond the gait and balance mechanisms—they include postural habits, the ability to compensate to physical stresses, and the growth of muscles, bones, ligaments, tendons, and other tissues. Normally, with each muscle contraction and relaxation, and every joint movement, important neurological patterns are created by the brain, just like with any memory. Shoes distort this process, and instead, the brain learns and designs irregular patterns of movement throughout the body.

In addition, other areas of the brain can be impaired. Normally, during early development in children, all the important neurological input from body movements trigger increased blood flow throughout the brain. This brings in oxygen and many other necessary nutrients to promote growth and development in areas that include learning, speech, and memory. Without the natural muscle contraction in the feet, for example, especially in the very small immature muscles that move the toes, impairment from wearing thick, oversupported modern shoes can reduce the brain maturing process.

In children plagued with posture- and gait-related problems, avoiding wearing shoes is even more important. This can help stimulate the above-mentioned neurological functions, which can, in itself, be very therapeutic. Rather than attempting the use of "corrective" shoes and related devices, such as inserts or braces, finding and correcting the causes, such as neuromuscular imbalance, is important.

Many physical ailments in adults could begin at this young age. Think about all the physical problems you've had in your life—it's possible that many began during development of the important brain-body mechanisms due to significant interference by shoes.

It seems silly to even be discussing the issue of children's shoes. Most people don't question the fact that eating junk food is bad for kids, or smoking cigarettes. The level of brain and body stress from wearing bad shoes can be just as damaging. The most logical, effective, and healthiest way for children to develop their whole body is by being barefoot.

Our Feet, Our Foundation

Most athletes don't have a fear of falling. Yet, we can all take a lesson from the *Leaning Tower*.

Galileo was said to have dropped two objects of different weights from the *Torre pendente di Pisa*—the Leaning Tower of Pisa—to prove his new theory that all objects fall at the same rate regardless of how much they weigh. In 1971, Apollo astronaut David Scott retested this theory from the moon's surface by dropping a hammer and a feather at the same time. While the moon's gravity is weaker than that of earth, the objects still fell about the same rate, albeit slower, hitting the lunar ground together.

While Galileo's use of the Leaning Tower for his research is probably a myth, he did develop the theory of objects falling at the same rate. But the Tower of Pisa is truly leaning because of the weak, shifting soil and the building's weak structural foundation; and the Apollo astronaut actually performed the gravity experiment, but mostly for NASA publicity.

The seven-story Pisa Tower, whose initial construction began in the twelfth century, began falling at some point during the building of its third story. This was due to a shallow foundation of only about 10 feet of unstable subsoil. For centuries, preventing the building's fall would be a topic of debate, study, and attempts at correcting the cause of the problem—and the focus was directed toward its faulty foundation. By 2008, after hundreds of tons of earth removal and other careful attempts at replacing and reconstructing the groundwork, architects and engineers finally said the Tower's unstable foundation was safe for the first time in history, at least for the next two hundred years. But the Tower still lists at just under four degrees.

The human body can be a lot like the leaning Tower: unstable and with a weak foundation. And the body's foundation begins with the feet. This means healthy, fit feet that can tolerate the downward pull of gravity, with muscles that are balanced, strong bones, good circulation, proper nerve activity that communicates with the brain, and other attributes including regular movement.

The feet must last a lifetime. The more you understand about the feet, the better you can care for them and even fix them when their function goes awry. The feet are subjected to more wear and tear than any other body part. Just walking a mile, you generate more than sixty tons—that's more than 120,000 pounds—of stress on each foot! Fortunately, and what's even more amazing, our feet are actually made to handle such natural stress. It's only when we interfere with nature that problems arise. Almost all foot problems can be prevented, and those that do arise can most often be treated conservatively through self-care.

From birth until death, your feet have a strategically important role in health and fitness. But too often, they become one of the most neglected parts of the body. If the feet lose their support—poor muscle function affecting the arches is a common affliction—the body can lean just like the Pisa, which in turn can lead to knee and hip problems, low back pain, spinal dysfunction, and other physical impairments. And an imbalanced body is more prone to tripping and falling down.

Your feet form the base of the body's physical structure, and any departure from optimal balance can have significant adverse effects not only locally in the feet but also for the entire body. These problems are often transmitted through the ankle, an extension of the upper part of the foot. Anatomists technically consider the foot and ankle as two separate areas, but I consider the ankle as a vital part of the foot for ease of discussion. The ankle is a vulnerable area; approximately twenty-five thousand Americans sprain their ankle each day. And probably many more develop at least one unstable foot and ankle.

Falling is also a common problem. Many people, including seniors, are not the same after a bad fall. It's often the start of a downward spiral set of related problems—the fall causes a knee bruise and pain, which produces weakness in the leg, and eventually, low back pain shows up, then spinal discomfort in the middle and upper back. It can be exhausting—physically, mentally, and emotionally. Too often, a bone fractures because bone density was poor or preexisting muscle imbalance was significant.

Poor function in the feet is one of the common causes of falling at any age. When the feet don't work well, there's usually associated muscle imbalance, poor posture, and distorted gait—all of which further the risk of a fall. You don't have to be a daredevil like a rock climber or downhill speed skier to fall. You can trip over a curb that is only several inches high and still get badly injured.

Reduced brain function also predisposes one to the likelihood of someday falling, even in people without severe cognitive or other physical problems. Those most vulnerable are people who have difficulty multitasking. For the distracted brain, the competing chores of thinking about sending an email to a friend, whether one has enough spinach for that favorite fish dinner tonight, and walking down to the basement freezer sometimes is too much to handle, and the risk of stumbling or falling down increases. Or, if you're working out with a friend or two, and chatting away, your posture may deteriorate, contributing to a fall.

Each year, millions of people fall. The problem is worse in those ages sixty-five and older, where about a third fall at least once. While about 80 percent of falls occur in this age group, 20 percent occur in those under age sixty-five. About half of those with a history of falling at least once will fall again in the near future. The Centers for Disease Control and Prevention (CDC) recently reported that, "Falls can lead to moderate to severe injuries, such as hip fractures and head traumas, and can even increase the risk of early death. Fortunately, falls are a public health problem that is largely preventable."

Prevention of falls is the best treatment. This starts with improved foot function. A well functioning aerobic system improves muscle function, gait, and overall balance.

Music can also help the brain with better balance and gait, lowering the risk of falls. In a recent study, Dr. Andrea Trombetti and colleagues of University Hospitals and Faculty of Medicine of Geneva, Switzerland demonstrated that listening to music as a therapy improved the brain's ability for a better gait and balance, significantly reducing the number of falls. Listening to music stimulates the rhythm centers of the brain, which impact physical movements.

The CDC also notes that:

- Among those age sixty-five and older, falls are the leading cause of injury and death. They are also the most common cause of nonfatal injuries and hospital admissions for trauma.
- In 2007, more than eighteen thousand older adults died from unintentional fall injuries.
- The death rates from falls among older men and women have risen sharply over the past decade.
- In 2009, 2.2 million nonfatal fall injuries among older adults were treated in emergency departments and more than 581,000 of these patients were hospitalized.
- In 2000, direct medical costs of falls totaled a little over $19 billion—$179 million for fatal falls and $19 billion for nonfatal fall injuries.
- Most fractures among older adults are caused by falls—the most common are fractures of the spine, hip, forearm, leg, ankle, pelvis, upper arm, and hand.
- Many people who fall, even if they are not injured, develop a fear of falling. This fear may cause them to limit their activities, leading to reduced mobility and loss of physical fitness, which in turn increases their actual risk of falling.
- Statistically, men are about 50 percent more likely than women to die from a fall, and women about 50 percent more likely than men to break a hip.

While the CDC and other healthcare establishments focus on recommendations such as getting an annual eye exam, making the home environment safer by reducing tripping hazards, adding grab bars and railings, and improving lighting, the feet are often responsible for falls. Poor foot sense and balance, which are intricately linked, can significant increase the risk of falling at any age.

In addition to falling, the feet help prevent many injuries in the knee, hip, low back, spine, and even the neck and shoulders. An important job of the feet is to help balance the whole body. The feet continuously communicate with the brain to regulate the rest of the body's daily movements, including standing, walking, and running, and even riding a bike. This is accomplished by powerful nerve endings at the bottom of your feet. These nerve endings are developed from infancy and their function is necessary throughout your life. Disturbances of these nerve endings due to trauma, disease, poor footwear, or neglect can lead to further health concerns.

The nerve endings at the bottoms of your feet also become a potential source of powerful therapy when properly and specifically stimulated. This approach can be used both preventatively and after some injury is realized. For example, a simple foot massage, even by an untrained person, can be great for your feet and brain because these nerve endings—also the reason it feels so good—are gently stimulated.

The Barefoot Bandwagon Blues

You know what I'm sore about? There are too many people jumping on the barefoot bandwagon. The *International Barefoot Running Day* is only a few short years old, yet humans were running barefoot long before there was ever an international observance. Nonetheless, millions of people—some reports put that number in the billions—took off their shoes on that fine day. That's not even counting those who don't have shoes. But it does include those who can't afford shoes, but buy them anyway. (Or those that steal them, but they probably don't take them off that much.)

There have been so many conditions that being barefoot benefits, supposedly. As it was once said, it cures what ails you. Certainly, at least, it fixes most of the injuries people have been continually getting since shoes went mainstream. Whether it's the zero-drop concept, the first metatarsal jam, wrecking your perceived exertion, using up more oxygen from their weight, shoes don't get much respect except from the people they hurt most.

I was browsing the medical library recently (I don't have a TV), and found an interesting study that measured the tension in the neck muscles as a result of wearing shoes. Those with higher heels had tighter neck muscles in the back. That was interesting, but not surprising. My first thought was that tight muscles in the back of the neck can be associated with weak ones on the front—the very pattern observed in whiplash injury. If you mention this study to a group of barefoot runners, they'll just shake their heads and say, "Oh, yeah, we knew that."

Some of the folks on the barefoot bandwagon are wearing minimalist shoes. Somewhere this has been deemed acceptable, except, of course, for the true barefooters.

So the barefoot bandwagon—the section underneath the back seat—is reserved for the minimalist shoe movement too. If we didn't have media, most people would not know about the minimalist shoe movement. I heard about it by word of mouth. I also heard some companies were just retrieving their high-inventory shoes that wouldn't sell and bragging about how good the company is to the earth for being on the barefoot bandwagon (at least, in the minimalist section). They are even allowed to call their products *barefoot shoes*. Now, *that's* interesting.

Of course, minimalist shoes also encourage many untold benefits. Why doesn't anyone ask the big companies, "Are the benefits of these shoes the cure for wearing all the other shoes you sell to people?" OK, now I'm getting a bit, well, nasty. Public companies that make shoes are not health care providers. They just sell shoes. They don't even really make them, people in other countries who don't have shoes do. I could hear the press conference now, by the marketing exec: "People choose to do with our shoes what they want. And if they get hurt from wearing them, it's their responsibility. Shoes don't injure people, people do." (Didn't the tobacco executives also make that argument?)

While I was browsing the medical library I saw another study whose title was in the form of a question (isn't that the purpose of a study—to *answer* the question?): "Is there an association between the use of heeled footwear and schizophrenia?" I doubled checked to make sure the Internet hadn't pulled a quick one on me, whisking me away to another site in the middle of a blink. But no, there were no flashing lights and screaming ads, all's quiet in the library.

Actually, there are scientists and other doctors who would answer "yes" to this question, based on certain evidence presented in other studies. This particular researcher is from Sweden, and he states that, "Heeled footwear began to be used more than 1,000 years ago, and led to the occurrence of the first cases of schizophrenia." He goes on to give some interesting explanations of this theory, including many references, and it was published in the prestigious journal *Medical Hypotheses*.

This researcher was persistent—many just go on to other topics once they get their paper published. Several years later, in another publication, this same author discussed other brain abnormalities associated with bad shoes. He states that, "The use of heeled shoes results in less eccentric contractions with decreased neurogenesis." He really meant to say that shoes impair the foot muscles, which in turn stimulates the brain less than with flat or no shoes, with the result that less brain cells are produced, injuring the brain.

If you mention this study to a group of minimalist wearers, and say that non-minimalist shoes can cause hallucinations, they'll shake their heads and say, "Ya, we knew that."

Yes, there is a barefoot bandwagon, and I've been ramblin' with it for a long time. But I still don't know who's driving.

There is much more to understanding great foot function. It can get complicated with details, especially when considering that we all have uniquely different feet—even on the same body.

But the most important component of this topic is also the simplest: being on your bare feet allows them to function better. Many people already know this and need to maintain that activity.

Others may require a form of rehabilitation I call barefoot therapy. This is discussed elsewhere and reviewed below.

10 Steps to Barefoot Therapy

Without exaggeration, I've spent most of my life barefoot—and I'm not counting the time spent sleeping. Though I never knew it until I studied the merits of foot muscles and biomechanics, I was performing the oldest natural remedy for my whole body—being barefoot. Looking back, I attribute my almost lack of physical injuries, despite being very active, to staying out of shoes. (There were the rare exceptions of a twisted ankle while running a rough trail or calf pain following a hard race.)

Being barefoot is perhaps the most potent treatment that helps the whole body maintain—or regain—the vigor and spring in its step. And, it's free. The best time to do it is right now.

Bad shoes of all types have infiltrated our closets, and wearing them has shamed our bodies into making irregular and erratic movements, increasing wear and tear on muscles, joints, ligaments and bones. It usually happens over a longer period of time so it's not as noticeable. The results are poorly functioning feet and an unhappy gait that creates back pain, knee and hip problems, spinal distortions, and even shoulder and neck dysfunction. It also reduces our balance, increasing the risk of falls.

Whether we're professional athletes or couch potatoes, most of us spend a considerable time on our feet, or at least we should. But if our foundation is not solid, flexible, and effective in moving the body above, we crumble over time like the Sphinx.

The barefoot and minimalist shoe movements are getting a foothold in mainstream articles and blogs of late. The once conservative publications, including *The New York Times*, are even including these topics, with whole books on the subject filling up Amazon's virtual shelves. McDougall's *Born To Run* was the breakthrough book because it brought a surge of acceptance to what was once a bunch of barefoot buccaneers.

But it's treading on trendiness, like the latest shoe fad. And when this happens, some of the more important, serious issues tend to be left right out of the discussions. The most important one of all is the fact that being barefoot is very therapeutic no matter who you are, and not just for the feet, but the whole body.

Of the dozens of therapies I used throughout my thirty-five-plus year career of treating physical injuries, from acupuncture and biofeedback to manipulation and exercises, being barefoot is one of the most powerful, easiest to apply, and quickest to get results.

Barefoot therapy has helped many people rehabilitate their feet—it's necessary because wearing almost all shoes, whether for sports, leisure, or dress up, can damage a foot's delicate muscles, nerves, and bones. By allowing the most natural of foot movements, being barefoot trains the feet to function better, and helps support the many structures above: the ankle, calf, knee, hip, back, and all structures up to the head. The result is that many aches and pains—including what some would consider chronic injuries like that bad hip or shoulder—get better.

But one cannot abruptly make the change to being barefoot after years of wearing dangerous footwear: those thick, over-supported shoes that ruin your feet have weakened your foot muscles. Whether you're wearing common running shoes with thick soles, high heels or most other footwear, weaning off them must be done at a pace that pleases your muscles—the weakest part of the average foot and the area most in need of rehabilitation.

No matter what your sport, if you're addicted to popular thick-soled trainers or just want to improve your running economy by wearing flatter, less supported shoes, or even run barefoot, the *transition* may take some time. The timeframe will depend on you. While a healthy body adapts to changes sooner, age, length of time in bad shoes, frequency of wearing new footwear or being barefoot, and other factors influence the process. Because making such a change will modify the gait, it should be done carefully and slowly over a period of weeks. In a recent study by Warne and Warrington ("Four-week habituation to simulated barefoot running improves running economy when compared with shod running," 2014) experienced runners in their twenties, who were used to wearing training shoes, were given Vibram Fivefingers to wear. They were allowed four weeks to slowly transition into training with them, with running economy tested on a treadmill before and after the four-week period. Running economy was no different between their thick training shoes and the Fivefingers, but after the four-week transition period economy increased dramatically, about 8 percent, as foot strike shifted more toward the forefoot.

Here are ten barefoot steps you can take to dramatically change your ailing physical body.

1. Take off your shoes. Don't put them on in the morning, unless you're going right outdoors, and when coming home, taken them off before walking into your house. Spend more time standing, walking, and otherwise being barefoot at home, in your office, and other indoor locations. It's best without socks, but a thin pair would be acceptable if your feet get cold. Walk on the bare floor, carpeted areas, and wherever your feet take you. This provides different types of foot stimulation to help muscles work better—the first step in rehabilitating your feet. And it's huge for the many people whose addiction to shoes is damaging the body. Do this for a couple of weeks before the next step.

2. Now, take the plunge and venture outdoors in your bare feet. This will provide additional foot stimulation over the comforts of home. Stick with smooth surfaces—your driveway, sidewalk, and porch. Do this for at least ten minutes. The different environment—the feel of new materials by your bare feet, including temperature changes—provides added foot stimulation. Do this in conjunction with step 1. A week or so of this additional activity and you're ready to move on.

3. Now venture off to uneven natural ground. Walking on grass, dirt, and sand will provide greater motivation for your feet to function better, helping the structures above be more stable. Start with just a few minutes if you're sensitive, but with three weeks of barefoot training, you'll be ready for this big step: work up to a short walk of about ten to fifteen minutes.

4. Most people will have to wear shoes for various activities—work, running, shopping, social occasions. During this rehab period, there are two important things to do with your shoes. First, start wearing thinner, simple footwear without supports. And second, make sure all the shoes you slip your feet into are a perfect fit. (I've discussed these two topic extensively in my books and on my website.)

5. Almost everyone can take these first four steps. It will help improve the body's mechanics from toe to head. But many people need more foot stimulus for additional rehabilitation. Being barefoot will do this eventually, but you can speed the process. Here's one way: a foot massage. A professional massage is always great, but you can treat your own feet daily at home, either by yourself or trading treatments with others. Even a five-minute massage for each foot can work wonders. Start with the feet relaxed, clean, and dry. A small amount of organic coconut oil is a nice option. Slowly and gently rub the foot all over using both hands, working up the leg where key foot muscles originate. Use firm pressure, but it should not be painful. Do this daily or as often as possible.

6. A key feature of optimal foot function is that it helps balance the whole body during walking, climbing stairs, running, and all other movements. Over time, wearing shoes can significantly diminish this balance mechanism. Being barefoot is very helpful, but here's a way to speed the process. You should be able to easily balance on one bare foot for thirty seconds or more. If you can't perform this action, it's probably due to foot dysfunction. Start

with attempting to balance on one foot for as long as you can, even if just for a few seconds; next, try the other foot. Balancing on each foot can gradually improve the communication between feet and brain promoting better balance throughout the body. Here's a way to incorporate this therapeutic activity into a regular routine: after a shower or bath—hold one foot up to dry it while standing on the other. Be sure to get each of your toes, and keep your foot relaxed. Then switch feet. Here's another good routine: each day when putting on your shoes, do it standing, holding your foot above your knee to put on the shoe and tie it, and then do the same with the other.

7. If you're on your feet a lot throughout the day, especially if you must wear shoes, you may get home with tired, sore, and hot feet. Cool them. A cold footbath can work wonders, even after a hot shower. It improves circulation, tones muscles, and improves overall foot function, and helps them recover from the day. Use a large enough bucket or foot tub that fits your feet without jamming your toes. Place your feet in cold water so they are completely submerged above the ankle. Add a small amount of ice to prevent the water from getting warm, but *do not* fill the tub with ice as this can freeze the foot, risking damage to nerves, blood vessels, and muscles. Keep your foot immersed for five to twenty minutes. A deeper bath can also cool the leg muscles. A cold footbath can do much more than an ice pack placed only on the area of discomfort. Take a footbath while answering email, catching up on phone calls, or use it as a time to relax and listen to music.

8. Sometimes, the use of a hot footbath can be therapeutic, not to mention comforting. Moist heat works better than a heating pad because it penetrates into the foot better. Use the same size footbath as mentioned above, and fill with hot water—not scalding—but most people can tolerate temperatures of around 90 to 100 degrees Fahrenheit. Adding Epsom salt (magnesium

salt) is also soothing. Beware: heat comes with contraindications. Do not use heat if you have an acute injury, especially one that's inflamed, swollen, or bruised; and avoid heat with any skin disorder, diabetes, circulatory problem, or an open wound. When in doubt about using heat, avoid it.

9. For many people, here's one more step: turn your outdoor barefoot walk into an easy jog or run. There are many ways to describe this process, but like other natural activities, your body already knows how to do it. Whether you begin on blacktop, smooth dirt, or other areas that are comfortable, as you naturally thicken the skin on the bottoms of your feet, you may be able to run anywhere barefoot. Use this barefoot time as a warm up for your longer run in flat shoes, a cool down, or keep it as a separate therapy. Many people take this as a launching pad for regular barefoot running, whether a forty-five-minute workout or even running in races.

10. This final step is most important, and for everyone. Once you've weaned off bad shoes, rehabbed your feet, and restored good foot function, be careful to avoid returning to old unhealthy habits by wearing bad shoes. It's that simple.

Rehabilitating your feet with barefoot therapy, and ridding the body of bad footwear, will bring renewed physical function. It can quickly bring back the spring and vigor in your step, prevent injuries, and help maintain overall physical activity for years to come.

MIND OVER MOVEMENT

Even before birth, our brains are busy preparing the body to be great endurance athletes. Newborns appear virtually helpless, but their brains are quickly creating 250,000 new cells a minute. While the infant can grasp well with their hands for very short periods, breathe sufficiently, nurse, and make erratic movements with the limbs, they don't appear very athletic. Yet the brain continues its pursuit 24/7.

The brain has an incredible incentive to move the body, relying on its natural, instinctual built-in *feed-forward* mechanism. This is essentially the mind sending messages to muscles instructing them to keep moving. This is so necessary and ingrained in the nervous system that movements even occur during sleep.

More movement stimulates greater brain growth, rapidly leading to additional and ultimately more coordinated efforts. The process continues at varying rates—aided by a barrage of sensory input that involves the natural *feedback* mechanism of the body sending massive amounts of vital information to the brain every moment. This continues the stimulation of more bodywide development, maintaining an ongoing astonishing neurochemical cycle.

The brain receives sensory input from the eyes, ears, skin, vibration, touching, and other senses, and from every square millimeter of the body, including muscles, ligaments, tendons, and joints. Even with each seemingly unpredictable, untamed, and inconsistent muscle contraction, the baby brain learns more ways to move, with the goal to accomplish these tasks in smooth, coordinated, powerful efforts and at greater speeds. The brain is continually teaching the body how to be a great athlete.

From the very first physical movements, muscle activity continuously plays a significant role in the development of a wide spectrum of brain function that also includes verbal communication, vision, sensation, and intellect.

Even the young brain remembers each and every body motion—a learning process that will continue throughout life. Other stimuli also play key developmental roles: seeing and hearing other people, sounds (especially music), blood sugar and other nutrients, oxygen, carbon dioxide, sleep, hormones, and much more. As muscle movement becomes fine-tuned, pushing the body to greater feats, there is a further expansion of the mind.

Tucked away in the brain is another piece of its complex puzzle. The autonomic nervous system involuntarily regulates day-to-day necessities such as heart rate, breathing, blood pressure, digestion, hormones, and untold numbers of other actions necessary for great athleticism.

As consciousness takes over more movement tasks, the body and brain improve and evolve. Now our young endurance athlete better understands the game. It's the meaning of training and racing—it's all about survival. The mind already senses the thrill of victory and the agony of defeat.

Nature knows that being the best is the only real option. The alternative is fatality. Of course, the young brain naturally wants to mature as fast and as complete as possible to accomplish this task.

A seemingly small organ, the brain is a mere 2 percent of the body's weight. Yet it demands 20 percent of the blood pumped by the heart, taking 20 percent of its total oxygen as well.

Starting at less than a pound, the brain only triples in size during the first twenty years. But it orchestrates the building of an athletic body that's some twenty to thirty times its birth weight. In a real sense, it's the interconnections of brain cells that help accomplish this amazing mission.

In the first five years of life, most of the brain's interconnections are created allowing the young athlete to make more sense of the world than most adults realize. Building to a hundred billion brain cells called neurons may seem like a lot. But the brain creates two hundred *trillion* (give or take) interconnections among these cells, with about 180,000 kilometers of nerve fibers making up the anatomy. This contributes to the creation of a unique individual athlete, despite losing thirty million brain cells each year due to normal wear and tear. (For comparison, our brain's two hundred trillion interconnections are more than the number of stars in our Milky Way galaxy—about four hundred billion. Astronomers estimate there are 170 billion galaxies in the known universe.)

All this activity is from a small glob of fat and protein—mostly water and biological tissues—that can fit in the hand. Its natural intelligence far outpaces today's artificial intelligence. And the brain adapts even to the most extreme conditions. (Consider an animal's broken leg, and how the gait is adjusted so the animal can continue moving and surviving. Or think about the surgical removal of half of a person's brain, and how the remaining part automatically rewires itself to make up for the missing parts, allowing the patient to live a normal life. This is an example of neuroplasticity.)

This period of a young athlete's life will be the most neurologically intense training time ever encountered. While the future sports world awaits him and her, the foundation of movement potential is already well established—that great gait is already hidden in the brain's network, gradually developing the body with this in mind.

Now, as the child's mind trains to creep, crawl, walk, and then run the hope is that nothing gets in the way.

At every stage of life, our continuously developing rebuilding body can run into problems—it can become impaired by various factors.

None of these amazing activities can continue without the presence of good quality food. Nutrition provides the building blocks for an excellent body made up of rapidly growing muscles, expanding brain, and everything in between—and at an astonishing rate. Food is the raw material used to make a whole new body—replenishing parts regularly throughout life.

No pain no gain can be instilled at an early age, such as when the sports announcer claims that "Big Joe is tough because he plays hurt." On the commercial break a cartoon character proclaims the greatness of sugar, while shoes of all types impair the body from the ground up.

These and many other obstacles can block the brain's natural progress to building the best athletic body, literally preventing forward motion.

For all athletes, it's not about finding the best training schedule, having a great race strategy, or trying a new sports diet. The brain already possesses this knowledge. The ability to train and race effectively already exists in a healthy brain.

Despite the vulnerabilities, we all possess resiliency. We recover, bounce back, and can even restore much of our youth through the process of becoming physiologically younger. It begins by building and maintaining a better brain.

Yes, everyone is an athlete. The more we progress, the longer we endure, and the further and faster we persist throughout the human race. Endurance, intuition and instincts are all entwined, and the sooner we allow them to flourish, the more athletic we become. It's not too late to continue the process, starting right now.

Don't Retire the Brain

I've been discussing the importance of the brain in sports performance since the 1970s, and was tempted to have a heading in this section called "Why the brain is important for athletes?" or some such title. However, the answer to that basic question is so obvious to virtually all athletes, not to mention anyone with an education that includes exercise physiology, so I chose to avoid it. However, to my surprise there continues to be a decades-old scientific debate about whether the brain is the primary regulator of training and racing.

Of course our brain is the most important part of us for every workout and race. Is there any doubt that the brain is the primary factor associated with the regulation of exercise performance? Sure, the heart is important, as is oxygen uptake, energy levels, and other factors, which the brain continually measures to monitor body movements. And, of course, the motor centers in the brain use this information to regulate each muscle contraction and relaxation producing that fine-tuned balanced gait we observe in great runners.

Of course, Dr. Timothy Noakes has been the prime proponent of the "central governor model," which he developed in 1998, about how the brain regulates training and racing. This model is based on sound science, yet others continue to claim that it's time to "retire" this idea.

For those interested in following this debate in the scientific literature—there are obviously a lot more interesting details than I note here—please read Dr. Noakes's article with references so you can read what his critiques say as well. You can find "Is it Time to Retire the A.V. Hill Model? A Rebuttal to the Article by Professor Roy Shephard" in the journal *Sports Medicine* (2011; 41 (4): 1-15).

Build Your Brain

We can actually build a better brain at any age. It's accomplished by doing more of the healthy habits that help us, while at the same time avoiding the harmful habits. Here are some important ways to do it.

1. **If We're Not Busy Being Born We're Busy Dying.**
   This is a paraphrase from the great singer-songwriter Bob Dylan. Presumably unaware of it, Dylan made a powerful neurophysiologic statement: By keeping our brains very active and fresh, we maintain high function. This means sustaining a high degree of sensory input and motor output, from a range of physical activity to regularly learning new things. It means challenging the brain's intellectual, emotional, and intuitive functions. In other words, never be bored and keep exploring.

2. **Keep Clear of Chronic Inflammation**
   The basic idea is simple—a bodywide inflammatory condition can significantly impair brain function both short and long term. Chronic inflammation is a common cause of most chronic diseases, along with many functional, subtle problems that can also reduce quality of life. This condition can also impair the *blood brain barrier*. Due to the inflamed blood vessels in the head, certain nutrients are unable to get into the brain. Choline is just one example, with low levels being associated with Alzheimer's disease. A simple *C-reactive protein* blood test can help monitor chronic inflammation. An important way to control inflammation is to balance dietary fats.

3. **Eat a Balance of Fats**
   Natural fats are a healthy part of a great diet. In addition to controlling inflammation, fat soluble vitamins, certain vital fatty acids, and other nutritional benefits make them essential. When using dietary fats (and oils) for cooking, use only olive oil, butter, or ghee ("drawn" or purified butter), coconut oil, or lard. Avoid all vegetable oil (such as soy, safflower, corn, and peanut), and trans fat (from margarine and other processed fats and oils). A common problem for many athletes is a low intake of the omega-3 fat EPA, which only comes from animal sources (the omega-3 fat in flax is poorly converted to EPA). Also avoid *trans* fats as they can replace the brain's healthy omega-3s. This topic

is complex, so please refer to other books for additional information on balancing fats.

4. **Avoid Eating Sugar and Flour**

This may be one of *the* most important lifestyle recommendations for a healthy brain. Sugar and processed flour (almost all that's in the marketplace) can injure the brain as quick as insulin is released (which typically begins during the oral phase of digestion). Likewise for other moderate and high glycemic carbohydrates—including other starches often used in packaged foods, and certain fruits like pineapple, grapes, and bananas. In addition to lowering blood sugar, insulin reduces fat burning, forcing the body to use more glucose, restricting its availability in the brain. While ketone bodies can be used for energy by neurons, their production is impaired by insulin too. Moreover, insulin strongly promotes inflammation. In addition, food frequency can help maintain optimal blood sugar levels, allowing the brain to have a constant supply of uninterrupted energy.

5. **Balanced Movement**

I'm a big fan of cross training. Of course, regular physical movement enhances locomotion, posture, independence, and other factors associated with quality of life, and it is a powerful brain therapy. Movement can significantly improve most if not all of the brain's areas including those associated with speech, vision, balance, memory, and even intellect. Even more potent is cross training. If you're a runner, cyclist, or other single-sport athlete, consider adding more movements in the course of the day and week, whether as separate workouts or other activities such as walking, working around the house and garden, and even regular dancing.

6. **Changing the Mind**

Like shifting gears in a sports car for better performance, a healthy brain changes consciousness frequently. While evaluating patients, for example, we may be in a *beta* state—very attentive and able to multitask on the many aspects of patient care. A relaxed and alert state is *alpha*. This occurs during downtime perhaps at lunch or when unwinding at day's end (or anytime when we have a spare few passing moments). *Alpha* produces very therapeutic effects for the whole body. While falling off to sleep, the brain drifts into *delta*. Unfortunately, too many people go there during the day, which is unnatural, unhealthy, or often harmful (since it can cause *human error* such as while driving a motor vehicle).

7. **Controlling Stress Hormones**

    Much of this book focuses on various physical, chemical, and mental stresses. By modifying training and footwear, diet, and better understanding many body mechanisms important for endurance training and racing, we can significantly reduce many stresses. The brain senses all stress to which we are exposed, and influenced by memories and emotions stored in nearby regions of the brain, responds immediately. This process begins in a small region of the brain called the hypothalamus. With its information about the status of stress, the brain directs the pituitary gland, housed in the middle of the brain, to produce a variety of hormones that are sent to the body for repair and rebuilding—essentially, adapting to stress. The pituitary releases hormones that stimulate the body's other glands, in particular those of the adrenals, to control metabolism, muscle function, and sex hormones, including testosterone, vital for healthy muscles. But when too much stress continues to bombard the brain, too many stress hormones are produced too often with the result of impairing the brain itself. Regulating physical, chemical, and mental stress is vital to maintaining a healthy brain for optimal training and racing, throughout life.

8. **Sleep All Night**

    Recovery from each day is critical for both the body and a healthy brain. This occurs during deep sleep. For adults, this means seven to nine hours of uninterrupted sleep each night. An unhealthy brain may be unable to accomplish this task. Excess cortisol (the stress hormone), blood sugar irregularity, physical impairments, and hormone imbalance are just some factors that can injure the brain, preventing it from regular rest. The accumulation of sleep deficit can maintain a vicious cycle that continually worsens brain function. While the brain doesn't really rest like the body during sleep, it's still essential.

9. **First Light**

Following a good night's sleep, waking up to daylight is the normal human circadian rhythm. But most people are exposed to sunlight later, when leaving the house. I recommend letting light into your eyes by looking outside. But glasses, contacts, windows, and sunglasses will prevent the normal light stimulation, so it must be done directly. Photosensitive cells in the eye also directly affect the brain's hypothalamus region, which controls our biological clock. This influences our brain to help maintain normal function—including hormone regulation, neuromuscular function, and behavior. Most cells in the body have an important cyclic pattern when working optimally, so potentially, just about any area of the body can falter without adequate sun stimulation.

Of course, there are more ways to improve brain function, which I've discussed in detail in other books and articles.

Can Music Make You More Athletic?

Yes it can—but not the way you think. Music can do many great things for the body. It can improve immunity, digestion, and even hormone balance. That could lead to better sports performance. Music can also help your muscles, and of course that can do wonders for any activity. But even more important is that music can improve brain function. And that, more than anything else, can definitely facilitate your ability to train and race better.

These are just a few of the favorite things music can do for the body. But there are other features of music that could ruin your running, biking, and other activities.

Athletes who turn on music for motivation might listen to "Eye of the Tiger" by the rock band Survivor (highlighted in the movie, *Rocky III*). This tune is so stimulating it has no doubt made more than a few couch potatoes take up sports. Likewise for "Chariots of Fire," the musical score for the film of the same name. Get up and go! But these and other physically motivating hits may get many going too fast, too far, or too often. These songs can get your heart pounding. In fact, it's possible that listening to these stimulating songs can raise your heart rate 10 to 15 beats a minute! That, of course, can lead to overtraining, which can trash your running because it wears you out.

Songs with enthusiastic driving beats are very popular in gyms, at races, and are often blasted during indoor workouts on the treadmill. But beware.

Beat music—those high intensity songs with strong fast tempos accompanied by loud thumping drums—can whisk us along, sprinting after some elusive pied piper. Power music like this can appear to make a boring workout exciting by passing the time quicker and stimulating our adrenal glands. Or give an early morning workout an extra dose of energy like a second (or third) shot of caffeine. But this is not why music can help endurance—this routine can do just the opposite. It can take you to where you don't want to go—to a world of overexertion that could lead to injuries, fatigue, and poor performances.

Just as important, it's best not to run with an iPod blasting through your earbuds (and certainly not during other events). While commercials have made this image sexy in our fast-paced overactive frantic society, it's not. If you need this much stimulation to get you going, there's something wrong. The joy and love of working out should be enough incentive, and the desire to get more fit.

Don't get me wrong, I love high-energy songs, and listen to them often. "Back in the USSR" (The Beatles) and "Dani California"

(The Red Hot Chili Peppers) are two that come to mind. I've even written some big beat songs (listen to "Twice in One Lifetime" on my website or online sites). But I've never listened to an iPod when running.

It's best to run without your iPod because you don't want to distract yourself while working out. In short, you want to better experience your body, and be more aware of how it feels. This is what natural workouts are all about. You want to sense each movement, every heart beat, your breathing. Knowing your body well will allow you to understand if something is not just right—much sooner than when your knee starts to hurt or back spasms sideline you.

Too often, as athletes get caught up in the stress of life, they look to a hard workout as a way to relieve the tension. But it doesn't really work that way. Adding tension to tension is a recipe for disaster. Along with the wrong kind of training, life's ongoing merry-go-round can put you in the ground, or at the very least, make you miss life as it passes. John Lennon said it best: "Life is what happens when you're busy making other plans."

Instead, you should get high. Training should be fun, peaceful, relaxing, and a time for pondering life or, as most of us know, just zoning out. It's what "runner's high" is all about. Often associated with natural opiates in the brain, or a cognitive state of dissociation, this so-called high has been linked with the same brain receptors stimulated by marijuana, which all humans possess.

While training is a common escape from the rigors of a busy daily life, anyone can train their brain to promote this conscious state even when not working out—once you learn it, you can click into it just about any time. This can really help your running. It has to do with brain waves.

When we're mentally and physically relaxed, unstressed, or doing something that takes us to our own private world, such as running, the brain goes into a unique conscious state marked by the production of alpha waves. This state can actually reduce high levels of cortisol. Listening to music does the same thing.

This is how music can help you run better—by listening when you're *not* running. By making it part of your life again, like when you were younger.

In this case, the brain gets many of the benefits, and since this part of the body regulates everything else, running improves too.

Every breath you take and every step you make is controlled by the brain. And when the brain is adversely affected by too much cortisol, running, like everything else, can become impaired. Too much cortisol can change the brain from goal-oriented learning and planning to habitual stimulus learning—you change from a proactive to a reactive personality. Not something that will help your running, or your life.

Too much cortisol can also contribute to conditions such as Alzheimer's disease, or in those without the condition, just bad memory even at an early age. It can both prevent the brain from forming new memories and keep it from accessing an existing one. Memory is something you want to keep—how else will you remember that great 10K or your first marathon? Paul Simon wrote: "Preserve your memories, they're all that's left you."

The better option is prevention. Reduce stress by ridding your life of junk (the physical, chemical, and mental types), and excess cortisol, add more music, and allow your body and brain to work better. *This* will help running.

Cortisol is one of our powerful stress hormones. It's powerful in two ways—good and bad. Its can help us out of a jam, whether it's sprinting down the street to get out of the sudden rainstorm while wearing formalwear, give us strength to lift a very heavy weight off our foot, or fight our way out of a jungle before being eaten by a tiger. These are all short-term needs for cortisol. But because we live in an intense pressure-pot of a world (one that we created), cortisol is often hanging around. What makes cortisol really bad is that it's there too much of the time, and when we don't really need it.

Since music can help by stimulating alpha waves, which can reduce high stress hormones, if you don't have time for music, it might just mean you *really* need it. Those who are too stressed usually don't have the patience for music, or if it is being heard, it's kept in the background. Or, there's just no place to put music in such a busy life.

If you're human, you love music. The earliest humans millions of years ago had music, and long before language developed. No doubt it was music that helped the brains of our ancestors develop language. Like every animal on earth, we all have music.

If you love music, you also need more of it because you know it will nourish your brain and body. And if you see music being played (the visual effect of video), it has additional benefits by stimulating more of your brain. It's even better when you play music (kinesthetics). And when you move the whole body to music with dance, it has an even greater therapeutic benefit.

Music can do more. It can balance muscles—those that are not balanced are usually the cause of physical problems associated with injuries, irregular gait, and poor running economy (using more energy and wear and tear than necessary).

Music can improve endurance, something all runners will welcome. By supplementing your life with music, and better regulating cortisol, you can burn more body fat, helping you run longer, and better. As a bonus, more fat is removed from storage, so it helps get you thinner. That's a nice thing.

Many athletes are so busy with their lives, surrounded by too much stress, that there's not enough time or energy for the relaxed alpha wave state. Instead, beta waves are more common—a state of consciousness that produces a very busy brain—thinking about all the things that need to be planned and done. It's too much thinking, and not enough relaxing. Your brain just can't stop chatting with itself. Sometimes it keeps you awake at night.

Training is a priority, so you make room for it. You don't let people interfere with your schedule, you wake up early or skip out of work to do it—you want it and need it. So do something healthy that will help your athleticism: create the time for improving it with music. Listen during mealtime, in the car, turn it on in the morning, have it on in the evening.

What types of music—classical or popular—can help your running? Which songs are best? The answer is easy: it's the same music that makes alpha waves, which is the music you enjoy most. So it's up to you to choose the tunes that will help your brain.

Still not sure which music? Consider these options. Think about what music moved you as a young person. Or, what song did you first fall in love with? Otherwise, if you don't know, you and your running need a real lot of help. Ask your parents for music suggestions—or your kids. Go to the music section of my website and listen to the songs and watch the videos. Borrow some CDs. Dust off your old record player and put on a vinyl album. Or just start buying or downloading songs.

But please don't turn on the radio. You may be listening to a good song one moment, then suddenly you'll hear the ravages of commercials, bad news, more commercials, and suddenly stress appears.

Brain Entertainment

Swimming, biking, and running in rhythm, and during all other physical activities, is an important component for improved performance.

A great athletic performance is usually one that is highly coordinated. While we think of synchronized swimming or figure skating as being highly rhythmic (like ballet, they are also performed to music), watching a cyclist racing through the Pyrenees, marathon runners in the lead pack, or a great swimmer gliding along the smooth open water is just as inspiring. The same is true for all other sports, when performed with the grace of a great gait. While we sense this coordination by observing the physical body, there is much more to it. The harmony of the whole physical and chemical body, from muscle movements to the throbbing heart and lungs, hormone actions and many others, are under orchestration by the brain.

It's called *entrainment*, the process whereby two or more interacting bodily systems work in a physiological harmony. I would add to that definition by saying *all* the bodily systems work together to create the greatest athletic performances. (The word *entrainment* may also refer to brainwaves, where one attempts to entrain their brain to get into a specific state of consciousness, such as alpha. Sometimes musicians talk about entrainment as being well connected with the music, getting into it, or in the moment.)

Entrainment is an evolutionary development associated with efficient movement that encourages better speed and endurance. Examples of entrainment in athletes including running in rhythm with the heartbeat, breathing rate, and muscle contractions, all while in step with the tapping of the feet's cadence. This coordination is a reflection of our natural built-in biofeedback mechanism. The most rhythmic athletes have the best body economy.

Impairment of entrainment can occur for many reasons:

- It could come from a physical illness, even a mild cold or allergy.
- A mental stress, including pain or anxiety.
- A muscle imbalance leading to poor joint movement.
- Impaired foot function, which may include wearing the wrong shoes.
- Improper equipment such as a bad bike set up.
- Swimming in a pool that's too short (too little distance to get into a good rhythm).
- Overtraining even in its early stage.
- Sometimes, seemingly innocuous habits like too much talking to a training partner during a workout, or listening to music that's not in synch with heart, lungs and stride can impair body rhythms.

Stride rate also affects the body's harmony, and stride length as well. This is one reason athletes go faster when they are in synch—in the example of running, speed is a function of the right stride rate and length for your particular body. Ideally, training at your own rhythm, and not following others around you, can help entrainment.

Those who are in synch can go faster at a lower heart rate. This is due to the fact that oxygen needs are lower with entrainment. While training in harmony, heart rate variability is improved (reduced), helping the autonomic nervous system—which, in addition to better performance can reduce the stress on the heart and lungs, help speed recovery, and allow fit athletes to be healthier.

If the body is not in rhythm, synch, balance, or whatever defines this natural harmony, one will not reach his or her athletic potential, be more prone to injury, and risk overtraining. When evaluating large numbers of athletes, I've found it's clear that those with efficient entrainment perform better, and those who learn to be more in synch improve significantly.

Along with gait and heart rate, studies also show entrainment can improve ventilatory efficiency. That is, for a certain number of strides, there is a breath. This is called *entrainment of ventilation and locomotion*, and it has been observed in cats, dogs, horses, jackrabbits, gerbils, rhinoceroses, wallabies, turtles, guinea fowl, alligators, and, of course, humans.

The synchronization of the body's components is well known. While day/night circadian rhythm is often discussed, this most human of patterns includes many individual patterns such as hormone cycles, intestinal function, brain waves, heart rhythm, and heart rate variability. It is all part of a complex but necessary organization of the body. We are most healthy when the body is in harmony, and athletes are more successful and less injured. It's no surprise that the brain manages the process.

Having only a great brain won't necessarily make you a great runner. Nor would just having the best body. But let them work in harmony, and running, swimming, biking, walking, and other movement can improve in efficiency resulting in better performance. Even without any change in training, keeping the body and brain synched will improve performance.

In human studies, the reported frequency of the link between breathing and striding has varied widely. (In fact, some researchers have found no evidence of entrainment at all.) Perhaps insightful, though, are the observations of Dennis Bramble and David Carrier at the University of Utah that the frequency of entrainment depends on the performance level of the runner. Experienced runners commonly coupled stride and breathing patterns very tightly. The most common ratio was 2:1 of strides and breaths, but at slow running speeds, this was frequently 4:1. However, in less talented runners, no synchronization of breathing and striding was observed at all.

This was evident in my evaluations with athletes, from beginners to world class. Those without entrainment were either slower or injured.

It's more than just the brain's motor center that tells muscle fibers to contract or relax, or the cerebellum's ability to add rhythm to movement. It's incorporating that coordinated rhythm with stride, heart rate, and breathing, for example, making everything synched like the instruments playing in a great band.

While an optimal stride length exists to minimize oxygen uptake, we can easily say the same about entrainment: it improves running economy.

My first experience with entrainment in athletes was working with professional dancers in the late 1970s, and soon I was spending considerable time on the track, observing runners of all ages, gender, and abilities. By the 1980s, as heart monitors were employed, it became evident that stride rate and length, gait, heart rate, and breathing were all coordinated. In faster athletes, these variables were more obvious, and in some people, this organization did not apparently exist.

I have written and lectured about this synchronicity for many years, and encouraged athletes to figure it out. Those who made the connection between heart rate or breathing, and stride, responded well to it by improving their performances. A common recommendation was to help athletes tap into this synchronous patter using breathing and foot strike. A simple example is breathing in for three strides, and out for the same number. This 3:1 relationship would change during a workout and race. A 5:1 pattern might exist during warm up and cool down, 2:2 during a competitive endurance event, with a 2:1 in the final "kick."

Similar relationships between body motion, breathing, heart rate, and many other mechanisms exist in virtually all sports. It is especially evident during swimming, cycling, and track and field events, but walking, yard, house, and office work—and most human—movement demonstrate it, even the movements of chewing our food. It also occurs at rest, where the heartbeats are in phase with breathing.

The synchronicity of the body was first measured and scientifically published in 1921 by Dr. Walter Coleman. In addition to measuring humans, he also evaluated a variety of animals, from cheetah and leopards, to bear and deer, with the same findings. More human studies followed, and by the 1950s most research was done in Germany. (These techniques may have been one of the so-called secret training techniques successfully used by East German and Russian athletes in the 1950s and '60s.)

While implementing these synchronization patterns into ones athletic training could sometimes work wonders, some had difficulty with it. Those who are musically perceptive have an easier time with it. The slower paced breathing rates make it easier to coordinate with foot strike, pedaling, or swim strokes. But for many athletes, the problem continued. In evaluating these athletes, the problem appeared to be in the cerebellum, the area of the brain responsible for rhythm.

If this is the case with you, the first consideration is to retrain the brain with simple biofeedback. This involves using a metronome—a small device that provides an audible beat one can adjust to the pace of physical activity.

Keep the Beat

While I don't recommend listening to music when working out, and in this case it's because you can't regulate the tempo, it's still important to keep the beat. So as an exercise therapy, use a simple beat best delivered with a metronome, which can be adjusted to an individual's changing pace through the workout.

In a recent study headed by Peter Terry at the University of Southern Queensland, Australia, researchers measured the effects of music on triathlete training. The results demonstrated that music's beat, more than its motivation, was important for improved performance.

Here are three simple steps to help improve brain-body synchronization. I recommend using breathing and foot strike during running, using strokes during cycling and swimming, and other patterns for your particular sport.

- *The Beat.* For many athletes, the brain's cerebellum, our rhythm center, is not highly coordinated. Some are not able to keep a consistent beat, or accurately tap their finger or toe to music. For others, dancing well is difficult or uncomfortable. In this case, the first step is to retrain the brain with simple biofeedback using a metronome. This small device provides an audible beat one could adjust to the paces of swimming, biking, and running. For example, while listening to the beating metronome, try coordinating each step with every beat. This may seem easy for some, but not for others—drifting offbeat is too easy, and can happen often. One should be able to adjust the metronome through the warm up, the main part of the workout, and through the cool down, adjusting the tempo to follow your footsteps. Employing a metronome for a period of time helps the cerebellum better coordinate movement—for example, by synchronizing one beat for each foot strike. Try it for a few weeks, making sure you can easily hit the ground (or whatever your sport) precisely with the beat. With a better ability to coordinate brain and body, the next step is to combine two systems.
- *The Two-Step.* A common recommendation at this stage is to count breathing instead of your metronome, and foot strike.

A simple example is breathing in for three strides, followed by exhaling for the same number. This 3:1 relationship would change during throughout a workout and race.

- *Shifting Gears.* Once you can coordinate breathing and footsteps, learning to shift gears is important. A 5:1 pattern might exist during warm up, which might change to a 3:1 or 4:1 while maintaining a steady state. During a competitive endurance event, it might shift to 2:2 with a 2:1 in the final finishing kick.

Because speed is a function of an economical stride rate and length for your particular body, training at your own rhythm, not that of another runner, can help entrainment and lead to better performance. While training or racing close to other athletes, you may inadvertently start mimicking their rhythms—try to avoid that.

Being in synch with entrainment can help you go faster at a lower heart rate. This is due to the combination of lower oxygen needs and a more economical gait.

Keep your brain busy—with balanced physical activity, give it great food, and mental, emotional, and other mind activities, and it will last a lifetime, bringing your body along for the ride.

THE MUSCLES THAT MOVE US

Thomas Edison once opined, "Great ideas originate in the muscles." The idea for a great endurance athlete is there too, as long as the brain is attached. Muscles don't move on their own so we really should refer to all the parts associated with activity—the neuromuscular system.

Muscles do much more than move us in millions of ways. Of course, I've discussed the fact that muscles burn both sugar and fat for energy. Here are some other important metabolic and other functions of muscles that significantly influence the athletic body.

- They play a key role in whole-body protein metabolism—amino acids help maintain protein synthesis in all organs, glands, and other tissues.
- They help prevent insulin resistance, metabolic syndrome, and diabetes—not to mention obesity and chronic disease.
- You'll get an additional source of energy from their amino acids (the liver can convert tyrosine, tryptophan, phenylalanine, threonine, and isoleucine into glucose, and leucine and lysine into ketone bodies).

- Important antioxidant function (in the aerobic muscle fibers).
- Important circulatory function (primarily in the aerobic fibers).
- They help the brain, playing a key role in vision, speech, intellect, and supplying the brain with a continuous and important sensory stimulation.
- Contractions provide the largest voluntary mechanical force on bones to increase bone strength and or mass.
- They help prevent osteoporosis, stress and other fractures.

Muscle loss is a serious problem in some athletes, especially during periods of detraining, and those over the age of around 60 years. Here are some factors associated with this condition (with more discussed in the section of aging athletes):

- In *healthy* aging there is no significant loss of muscle mass or function.
- Sarcopenia—the loss of muscle in aging—exists in about 30 percent of those over 60 years.
- Chronic inflammation and poor diet (especially low protein) are significantly related to muscle loss. (*Cachexia* is the extensive loss of muscle mass, strength, and metabolic function associated with chronic disease.)
- Muscle loss reduces quality of life, increasing frailty, risk of falls, loss of independence, and the high rate of institutionalization.
- Muscle loss is a serious problem in retired or injured athletes.
- The key to muscle loss is prevention. This can be accomplished by:
  - Remaining fit and healthy.
  - Maintaining hormone balance (testosterone, estrogens, growth hormone, and all others.).
  - Avoiding excess stress (high cortisol).
  - Maintaining adequate vitamin D status (getting enough sun exposure).
  - Maintaining adequate protein intake.

In addition to influencing many health factors, muscles obviously control movement, from lying, sitting, and standing posture to gait and all actions of the body. While I can go through the whole body and systemically explain why each muscle is so important, including how each affects others, I won't. One important example I will highlight is the abdominal muscle—an extensive group that plays various and diverse roles for the athletic body.

The Abdominal Muscles

This extensive group of muscles, in both attachments and functions, may be the most misunderstood of all.

When it comes to movement, nothing is more important than the abdominal muscle group. At the core of their function are diverse fibers that attach on the front, sides, bottom, and back of the trunk, from the midsection down to the pelvis. Not only can these muscles flex, extend, laterally bend, and rotate the trunk, the abdominals can help move the pelvis, thigh, spine, head, and neck. They are also vital for proper breathing, and physically protect the intestines. But great abdominal muscles are more than what you look like in the mirror.

In addition to their wide ranges of movement, these muscles play a key role in stabilization. Even before we engage the arms and legs for a run, walk, swim, or other activity, the abdominals must first contract to create a firm foundation. The brain, which manages all muscle action, plans ahead by stimulating the abdominals to assure a stable enough body for follow-up activity that is also efficient and safe.

The abdominals attach, via tendons, to various bones—ribs, sternum, and pelvis—and to many soft tissues including other muscles and fascia. This contributes to the movement of additional body areas, such as the shoulders and hips. In the abdomen, good muscle balance helps prevent the development of different types of hernias, including inguinal, femoral, hiatal, rectus, and umbilical.

Dysfunction of the abdominals is a common cause of posture and gait irregularities, muscle imbalance, and related back, neck, pelvis, shoulder, and other injuries. Practitioners, trainers, coaches, and others often assess these muscles through observation (watching a person walk or run), an oral history (such as asking, "what movement is most and least painful"), and muscle testing (simple biofeedback). Only rarely is high-tech evaluation, such as MRI, necessary.

The abdominal muscles include various components:

- The rectus is on the front and either side of the midline.
- The transverse makes up the deeper layers on the front and sides.
- Both the external and internal obliques are on the sides of the abdomen.
- The very small pyramidalis is located in the middle of the lower part of the abdomen, in front of the rectus (and may work with the pelvic floor muscles).

From the brain, the nerves that control all these muscle fibers exit through a large number of spinal vertebrae—from the 5th to the 12th thoracic area.

Contraction, relaxation, and actions associated with muscle control can be complex. But during natural activity, a single muscle does not usually work in isolation but in harmony with others, not unlike an orchestra with individual instruments that must play just at the right time. Physical activity involves a nearly infinite number of variations all regulated by the brain.

Instead of attempting to isolate an abdominal or other muscle in a workout, such as with tradition sit-ups, it is best to create natural activity for activation of more muscle fibers. An example is lifting a heavy weight off the ground, especially when bringing it up to the waist, chest, or above the head. These actions activate many muscles in a more balanced way, including all the abdominals.

Virtually all actions involve the abdominal muscles to some degree—from biking, running and walking, to swimming, swinging a golf club, and playing chess. Even when the body is at rest, the abdominals help keep it stable and balanced.

Despite the hype, the abdominals don't bulk up nearly as much as other muscles because they are relatively thin structures. Those with so-called six-pack abs look that way to a large degree because of low belly fat, showing muscle detail very well. But reducing this fat won't happen by performing sit-ups—spot reducing is a myth. Burning off body fat is best accomplished by improving the metabolism, where diet plays a dominant role.

Sit Up Stress

Modern society has created many so-called luxuries like cushiony sofas, chairs, and car seats, which render the abdominal muscles less active. The result is the common bulging belly (although much of this problem is excess fat), muscle imbalance, back pain, and other physical problems. Taking advantage of this dilemma is a hyped-up industry marketing expensive abdominal exercise equipment. And most of these workouts don't work well and can even create other imbalances since they don't stimulate all abdominal fibers. Likewise for popular sit-ups.

Performing traditional sit-ups learned in gym class usually won't help because of limited action, not contracting nearly enough abdominal fibers. In fact, this routine sometimes worsens fitness as evidenced in the exacerbation of low back tightness and even pain in many individuals.

Developing all the abdominal muscles means stimulating those associated with multiple movement including flexion, rotation, extension, and lateral bending, both in the lying and upright position. A great abdominal workout is swimming with different strokes on your back, while face down, and sideways. This can play a more important role in development than traditional sit-ups because you can contract the full spectrum of muscle fibers.

For the few who truly need more abdominal power, which includes those athletes in boxing, martial arts, football, and other contact sports, but usually not endurance, performing "crunches" can help. Lying on your back with knees bent to ninety degrees, sitting up thirty to forty-five degrees only, then slowly back down. Reverse crunches, where the pelvis is lifted off the floor, encourages even more lower muscle contraction. Adding rotation, lateral bending and other actions, including stimulation of the pelvic floor muscles as described below, can help even more. But don't perform these to the point of any significant fatigue—soreness should not exist the next day. Enlisting the help of a professional to properly learn these or other effective routines is best.

The Optimal Abdominals

Not everyone has poor abdominal function. But there is a good chance that part or all of this muscle is impaired if you have back tightness or pain, poor posture, irregular gait, or have injuries in areas influenced by these fibers. And, if you have been unsuccessfully toning your belly, you may have neglected too many abdominal fibers while overworking others.

Below are two easy-to-implement activities that can significantly help improve abdominal muscle function.

- The first is a natural biofeedback therapy, great for those just starting to get into shape, people with back problems, and many others, including athletes who have indications of abdominal dysfunction. While lying comfortably on your back, place the hands on the mid-abdomen and slowly breathe in and out. Feeling the belly push out on inhalation and pull in during exhalation is the basic breathing mechanism. If you are not able to perform this simple action easily, or especially if you breathe backwards, just practicing the movements two or more times each day for a few minutes can significantly help the abdominals (and diaphragm) function better. This activity is part of a great relaxation technique called "The 5-Minute Power Break" that can help balance many muscles, reduce stress, improve breathing, and enhance brain function.

- The second activity involves a combination of forced exhalation, pelvic floor muscle activation, and varying ranges of motion. This can be done lying on your back or standing, and eventually you will be able to perform them in any position. Here is the process:
  - Blow air out of the lungs; and then force more air out through contraction of additional abdominal fibers.
  - Be sure to activate the transverse abdominals, an often-neglected part of the group, which encourages contraction of the pelvic floor muscles. Place your hands on the sides and lower most part of the abdomen to feel them tense up.
  - At the same time, tighten your pelvic floor muscles. If you're not sure how to do this, think about stopping the flow of urine. (These are the muscles stimulated during Kegal exercises for incontinence and sexual dysfunction.)
  - Even more abdominal contraction will occur when your belly button is strongly pulled inward, as if it is trying to touch the spine.
  - As you are able to perform all these actions, begin adding various movements—left and right rotation and side bending, flexion, extension, and combinations. This will help develop the full range of abdominal muscles.

Many people can benefit from performing this routine regularly to help retrain unused abdominal fibers. In a short time you will be able to use these muscles at other times:

- Before getting up and down from lying and sitting positions to avoid over-tightening the back.
- While sitting to counter the physical stress of this position.

- When bending to maintain stability.
- Just prior to lifting objects for added support and strength.
- While standing to maintain a better posture.

As you consciously use this natural biofeedback action, it will become easier for the brain to utilize more of the abdominal muscles (and more fibers) when the need exists, which is much of the time. Ultimately, you may not even be aware of how much contraction is taking place. This activity is especially important while working out to maintain a better gait and protect joints, bones, and other tissues from injury. Improved abdominal muscle function can also enhance athletic performance.

Pain Control

Poor abdominal muscle function can significantly contribute to common pain syndromes. If your back, neck, pelvis, hip, or other area is hurting, try this simple activity:

- Stand barefoot looking straight ahead, with feet spread about shoulder width.
- Perform the abdominal biofeedback movements described above with forced exhalation, belly button back, and contraction of the pelvic muscles.
- While the abdominal muscles are contracted, avoid holding your body too rigid—maintain a relaxed support. Even though you obtained this position with forced exhalation, now you can breathe normally while keeping the body firm.
- For most people, performing this simple routine can reduce—often eliminate—pain immediately. Learning to maintain the necessary support from the abdominals can keep pain away.
- Once the abdominal muscles are better able to contract as needed, the brain can more easily correct other imbalances that cause pain.

If you have pain while moving, perform the same procedure. Stimulate abdominal contractions while walking, running, swimming, biking or during any activity. Improving gait through better muscle function can reduce pain and make movement more efficient.

Muscle Dysfunction

Like other muscles in the body, abdominal dysfunction can occur for two main reasons. First, the muscles may lose tone, or strength, from disuse, even in athletes. Too much sitting is a common reason, even in athletes. Well intentioned but poorly designed exercises, such as traditional sit-ups or a single ab machine, can result in muscle imbalance, resulting in some fibers that are too tight while others stay weak.

The result is poor posture, altered gait, and tightening of the antagonist muscles, especially those of the lower back. This is the clinical picture in most patients with back pain. But just contracting the abdominals sufficiently and regularly in the course of the day as described above can significantly help improve muscle function and reduce or eliminate pain.

A second cause of abdominal muscle dysfunction is the condition of *abnormal inhibition*. This is a neuromuscular problem that includes the brain and nerves connecting to each muscle fiber. In this situation, the same type of low back pain or other problems can develop. But exercise won't help much as this is caused by the nervous system, not disuse or true weakness. It is as if a "circuit breaker" was tripped, turning off the muscle. A healthy body can sometimes correct this problem. But often, finding the right therapist who can properly evaluate the muscles and apply the appropriate therapy may be necessary.

To address the needs of both situations—poor strength and neuromuscular dysfunction—simple biofeedback can be effective. This helps train the brain to better communicate with more muscle fibers during each contraction resulting in better function and increased strength. (See Manual Biofeedback.)

The abdominal muscles may be our greatest fitness friend. Proper care involves using them wisely—don't avoid or abuse them. Retraining communication between the brain and muscle is easily accomplished and maintained, and can result in better body function, elimination of pain, and improved athletic performance.

Abdominal Addendum

This topic always brings many questions. People are often too sensitive about their abdominal muscles, and many ask about low back pain and abdominal muscle tone.

While traditionally, the notion that tightness in the lumbar spine is due to poor abdominal function, there is much more. Recall that muscle imbalance is the combination of weakness and tightness, often with associated pain. This is the common condition of poor functioning abdominals with low tone, and back muscles that are too tight. But tightness can occur all the way up the spine into the neck, as well. So mid- and upper-back pain can also be caused by weak abdominals.

In addition, the abdominals have an important synergistic relationship with the muscles in the front of the neck. Poor abdominal tone can result in tight and painful muscles in the back of the neck, and even those in the head and shoulders. This is especially common in people who sit too much.

While weak and tight muscles may hurt, those imbalances can also create joint pain. There are many joints throughout the spine and pelvis, and if poor muscle balance exists, improper joint movement follows leading to inflammation and chronic pain.

No-Name Technique

Many techniques and systematic methods can improve abdominal muscles and overall body function. I won't comment on each one other than to say they can all have value when applied properly. However, an important point is that conscious awareness of abdominal action—being able to feel the muscles contract and retrain them as needed—is vital to improving the function between brain and body, thereby allowing the abdominal muscles to perform their job whether you are aware of them or not.

Walking-Running?

Many people are surprised to read that walking and running can help tone the abdominals. Neglecting belly tone, which renders these muscles less active during any movement, is a common problem. But those who use the abdominals more in day-to-day movement also contract them during walking and running. A recent study showed that triathletes who use their abdominals due to natural cross-training activate these muscles more while running compared to runners who don't cross-train.

Vocalizing

The abdominal muscles also play a key part in communication. Both vocalization—simple talking—and singing are best performed standing. In this position, the abdominals can flex the trunk for more effective breathing and body language, resulting in better tone, power, and pronunciation.

Abdominal Testing

Like most other muscles, an important way to evaluate the abdominals is manual testing, although it is not easy to isolate each part. While evaluating their function, the same stimulation of contraction provides a simple way to treat them through biofeedback. This can increase their overall function and strength.

The Myth of Core Muscles

The above discussion of abdominal muscles is all about the body's central balance. It also involves a lean waist. These factors are the real core of a balanced body.

When most people hear the word "core," thoughts of grueling strength sessions, sweat, and six-pack abs come to mind. Many think that so-called core muscles are comprised only of anaerobic fibers and the abdominals, and bulking them up is how to have a great looking, sexy power core. Workouts include crunches and sit-ups, with a bunch of weights thrown in, all with a high-rep, fatiguing approach, the 48-hour rest, then doing it all again.

Most of this is either wrong or unhealthy. Let's look at the big picture, better terminology, and a definition.

Core Is Out

The once tidy little name was a great marketing tool, but is now connected with communication breakdown. It's too restrictive, a vague and confusing term, and without sufficient consensus. *Central balance* refers to the muscular control of the entire trunk. Impairment here can be the cause of many types of injuries throughout the body.

Another central issue is a lean waist. Too much stored fat, especially in and around the abdomen, poses serious health and fitness consequences.

Two of the most significant abnormal findings common in the world today are poor central balance, and an overfat abdomen. These problems are often related, and always serious. Both affect posture and gait, contribute to spinal pain, foot and knee problems, and many other exercise-related injuries. And both usually have metabolic consequences too, including lower energy, chronic illness, and increased body fat. I will discuss each below.

Central Balance

When standing up straight, a balanced body's center of gravity is in the pelvis, just in front of the sacrum (the bone that connects the bottom of the spine to the two large pelvic bones). But this central balance point is always changing, sometimes drastically, because we move so much. The muscles in the trunk, under control of the brain, control these changes and regulate central balance.

Let's better define our central body, without seeming too simplistic. Our anatomy is primarily composed of a) a central component, and b) all the rest:

- The central component is the trunk, our hub, whose functional parts include the abdomen from chest to pelvis, and the back from the bottom of the neck down to the pelvis. It includes the sides of the trunk, too, and more than just the main outside muscles, the abdominals and sacrospinalis. Deeper muscles such as the psoas are just as important. Our hub plays a vital role in stabilization and movement, maintaining proper posture and gait, and protecting organs, glands, and nerves (including the spinal cord). The central body's many potential motions help coordinate the arms, legs, and neck to move well.
- In the rest of the body, our arms, legs, and neck attach to the central part like tentacles sensing the world. Our feet feel the ground to better propel us, and our fingers sense the environment above. The information received is sent up through the neck and into the brain.

Central balance refers to the optimal stabilization and movement of the body's trunk. Among the muscles accomplishing this are a key trio that includes the abdominals, psoas, and sacrospinalis.

- The importance of the abdominals was discussed above. These muscles wrap around the trunk, from front to back, to create unlimited movement potential, along with stability so our arms, legs, and neck can move effectively.
- The psoas is a large muscle connecting to the discs of the lower six spinal vertebra, and then traveling through the pelvis attaching to the inside front of the femur (thigh bone) just below the hip joint. The actions of this muscle are wide-ranging and include flexion and lateral bending of the trunk, extending the low back, and flexion of the hip/thigh forward. It also outwardly rotates

the leg, influencing placement of the foot and ankle during gait (and, when unbalanced can contribute to excess pronation). The psoas, an important stabilizer of the low back, pelvis, and hip, usually work together with the iliacus muscle, and together are referred to as the iliopsoas.

- The Sacrospinalis (also called the erector spinae) is comprised of a large group of smaller back muscles on either side of the spine. They attaché on the vertebra and ribs and from the pelvis to the head. This muscle extends the back, laterally bends it, and is important for many spinal movements. Like the abdominals, the sacrospinalis greatly assists in stabilizing the central body from behind so other muscles above and below can better perform their actions.

Stabilization and movement of the trunk is an ongoing action, one that requires endurance. The muscle fibers performing this task are the aerobic ones, with anaerobic ones used when quick, short actions are necessary.

All the factors associated with strength and neuromuscular balance applies to both the psoas and sacrospinalis. In review, just strengthening these muscles does not guarantee they will function properly as impairment may be due to the brain's control over them. In addition, stretching these muscles can be harmful, too (see Update on Stretching).

Overall, the most common pattern of imbalance in this trio of muscles is as follows:

- Weakness or poor strength of the psoas.
- Weakness or poor strength of the abdominals.
- Tightness of the sacrospinalis.

In the common scenario above, the psoas and or abdominals usually weaken, causing secondary tightness of the sacrospinalis. When this situation exists the most common symptom is pain, typically in the low back, but also in the groin, hip, pelvic, or other areas. The most common sign is imbalanced posture and gait as these muscles are vital for smooth movements whether walking, running, biking, swimming, or anything else.

Of course, any combination of problems is possible in given individuals. Most important, one should have good balance between these three muscles because they play a significant role in our central balance. Even minor muscle impairment can have devastating consequences anywhere in the body, from head to toe.

Central Fat

Call it a beer belly, love handles, or just a widening waist. Too much trunk fat is worse than it looks. Clinically, too much abdominal fat is called central obesity. With a worldwide overfat epidemic, no one is exempt from this problem, including many athletes.

While "spot reducing," such as performing sit-ups to lose belly fat, is a popular trend, it's one that is never truly successful. To lose central body fat the cause of the problem must be addressed.

Perhaps the most common cause of excess central body fat is refined carbohydrate consumption. This occurs because of insulin's role in converting up to half the refined carbohydrates one consumes into stored fat.

Increased belly fat is a serious sign of poor health. It's commonly associated with heart disease, Alzheimer's, cancer, diabetes, and chronic inflammation. The problem is seen in those with chronically high stress hormone, cortisol, and high blood fats (triglycerides).

Increased belly fat will not only stretch your pants size, but also stretch the abdominal muscles, too. The lengthening causes them to weaken, triggering the sacrospinalis muscles in the back to tighten. This is a popular recipe for chronic low back pain and disability. This also alters gait and can interfere with exercise at any level.

Of course, other central muscles are important. These include the diaphragm, *latissimus dorsi*, *gluteus medius*, and *maximus*, the mid and lower *trapezius*, and others. The fact is, all the body's major muscle are vital for overall balance. But, significantly, more people have imbalances in the trio of muscles described above.

By being both healthy and fit, and sometimes with the help of an appropriate healthcare professional, correction of these problems is possible (see Muscle Imbalance). The problem of excess of abdominal fat is relatively easy to remedy—avoid eating refined carbohydrates, including sugar (see The Two-Week Test).

A better understanding of our body's central balance, and the avoidance of too much stored fat, can dramatically improve overall health and fitness.

Muscle Fatigue

Anyone who has ever competed knows the feeling of muscle fatigue. You want to keep going at the same pace but can't. The mind is willing but the body is weak. Power output cannot be maintained. Even inactive people know the feeling after some hasty yard work. While a certain level of muscle fatigue is normal with physical activity, too much can impair training, reduce health, and ruin your race.

There are generally two types of muscle fatigue:

- Mild to moderate fatigue does not result in soreness or cause imbalance in muscles.
- Excess fatigue causes soreness, leads to muscle dysfunction, and is often associated with overtraining.

When a single muscle is evaluated, fatigue can be measured as a reduction of power. In the case of the whole body, it is slowing down the pace during running, cycling, swimming, or other activity, all while the heart rate remains the same or is elevating. Managing muscle fatigue is an important aspect of effective training, one that contributes to improved performance. The process begins by understanding the normal, abnormal, and origins of fatigue.

Normal and Abnormal

In the natural state, mild and moderate muscle fatigue is normal and even necessary. Proper training means working the body and its muscles a bit harder than usual—a state called *overreaching*—and then allowing adequate recovery. When properly done, the body learns to accomplish more work with the same effort. In other words, we get faster at the same heart rate. (When this does not happen, it means imbalance is preventing progress.)

While normal, healthy fatigue encourages muscles to better adapt and prepare for more power, there are other benefits. Included is improved heart, circulation, and lung function; enhanced regulation of oxygen and carbon dioxide; better utilization of muscle energy; and optimal metabolism of lactate. The most important end result is a better brain, one that can best manage all the body systems leading to greater athletic performance.

When the delicate balance of work and rest is disturbed, normal fatigue turns abnormal and problems arise. Too much intensity or higher volume training can cause undue, *excessive* muscle fatigue because we go outside overreaching, into that zone where muscles are damaged. While this occurs during and after a race, making proper recovery a necessity, it can happen more regularly with imprecise workouts, or following a program not specifically designed for our particular needs.

Working out this way presents several problems. We build a "debt" of muscle fatigue, whereby training exceeds the body's ability to properly recover. It can eventually lead to injury or ill health, although just one fatiguing session that is damaging enough, especially without appropriate recovery, can impair health. As the problem escalates we may pay the penalty of poor performance on race day because muscle fatigue still exists. The same dilemma occurs when racing is too frequent, there is inadequate taper, recovery is too short, or a combination of factors.

These two types of muscle fatigue—normal/healthy, and abnormal/harmful—are best exemplified in strength training. When performing most weight programs of several sets of high repetitions, muscles are isolated and worked to the point of failure, which means significant fatigue. The muscle can no longer lift the weight. This is traumatic, and the body's response is to produce stress hormones. The need for recovery is significantly increased—something many people don't obtain. The next workout, whether easy or hard, typically starts before one is properly recovered. What is the alternative?

A healthy option is to perform less repetitions and sets, and avoid excess fatigue. A single set of strength training, for example, is as effective as three sets for increasing strength. Because muscles are not significantly damaged, added benefits include faster recovery, the strengthening of bone, stronger muscles without bulking up, more fat burning, and no impairment of aerobic function.

Damaging Fatigue

Excess fatigue is often glorified as part of the "no pain, no gain" work ethic in today's social sports world. While some athletes, such as those in track and field, power lifting and football, get closer to the line of overtraining and are injured more easily, endurance activities are much different. Running, biking, swimming, and multisport events rely mostly on aerobic training, which, when properly done, does not produce significant muscle fatigue unless the *volume* of training increases too much. Despite this, improvements in performance should regularly occur—in other words, swimming, biking, and running at faster paces at the same heart rate during training and racing.

Excess muscle fatigue is also associated with other problems:

- Fatigue generated by an intense workout can increase stress hormones and potentially impair endurance.
- A muscle that is fatigued will not contract as many fibers, reducing power and increasing weakness.

- Muscle fatigue can impair associated joint movements (such as quadriceps and knee joints), and contribute to such chronic conditions as osteoarthritis.
- Poor posture and gait irregularity result from muscle fatigue. This problem can last many hours following training or racing.
- Working a fatigued muscle can lead to muscular imbalance and result in further damage to ligaments, tendons, joints, fascia, or bone.
- A fatigue-producing anaerobic interval track workout, like a popular weight-lifting session, requires significant recovery—at least 48 hours, often more, before working out again.
- Muscle fatigue can significantly reduce training and racing performance.
- During competition, varying one's speed can cause more muscle fatigue compared to racing at a steady-state pace.
- Respiratory muscles can often fatigue, sometimes more than leg muscles, and limit maximum exercise intensity and duration. (This is associated with the relationships between inhalation and exhalation, and gait and foot-strike.)
- Muscle fatigue can result in metabolic disturbances, including the over-accumulation of ammonia from protein breakdown. (Taking branched-chained amino acid—BCAA—supplements can worsen this condition.)
- Equilibrium can become disturbed with muscle fatigue. Poor balance can lead to inefficient movements and increase the risk of trauma (such as crashing a bike or twisting an ankle).
- Muscle fatigue can worsen symptoms in those with chronic fatigue syndrome, fibromyalgia, and chronic pain.
- Anaerobic muscle fibers fatigue much more easily and quickly, while aerobic fibers are relatively fatigue-resistant.

Causes of Muscle Fatigue

While there may be many reasons for muscle fatigue, through the years a variety of trends have pinned the blame on the "usual suspects," as if the answer to the age-old question has been found. These include cardiovascular limitations, oxygen deficits, lactate levels that change pH, diminished muscle energy, and others. Any or all of these common issues may contribute to muscle fatigue, but not as a primary factor.

Muscle fatigue is usually countered with energy issues. Our muscles use both fat and sugar (glucose) to create ATP, the ultimate source of energy for muscle contraction. Currently, the popular notion is that when ATP falls below the muscle's ability to contract, we become exhausted. If local energy levels were the primary reason for muscle fatigue, it would just be a matter of gulping down enough sugar during a race to keep going. But as studies show, muscle energy usually remains more than adequate even after a long, intense effort. This is the reason most athletes have a "kick" at the end of a grueling race. Despite the fatigue that occurs during the event, there is almost always a seemingly newfound ability for the muscles to work much harder and quicken the pace in the final segment of an event.

Other popular notions about muscle fatigue have included limitations of the cardiovascular system—the lungs to bring in oxygen and the heart to circulate blood to the working muscles. Associated with this is the obsession of VO_{2max}—a number athletes love to toss around despite serving no practical purpose.

Another culprit is said to be lactic acid, where changes in muscle and blood chemistry, a rise in pH, impair muscle function leading to fatigue. For decades, products proclaiming to "neutralize" these exercise-impairing metabolites are found in pop magazines and store shelves. They don't work. As we now know, lactate is an important metabolite and, in fact, an important energy source.

These theories proclaiming *the* cause of muscle fatigue do not make sense—just consider that if the levels of oxygen or ATP fall below the level necessary for muscle contraction, or lactate levels rise too high, an athlete would not only slow down but also stop performing, and even collapse, since muscles would be unable to maintain a standing posture.

Fatigue can also be discussed from a standpoint of peripheral versus central. In other words, what happens in an individual muscle versus the big picture?

Avoiding excess muscle fatigue should be a key goal of training and being healthy. Recovering from it before a race can result in greater performances. But cunning public relations campaigns have brought us lines of nutritional supplements that supposedly gives us what a great diet won't, pharmacologic compounds that cover symptoms of fatigue, and physical items such as bad shoes supposed to give us energy, all aimed at an athlete's feelings and emotions. And they are successful as millions of people will go to the extreme to improve performance.

Build a Faster, Fatigue-Resistant Body and Brain

Almost everyone feels muscle fatigue. Normally, it can be noticed during a race, hard training session, or a long workout. But if pushed too much we feel the consequence of *excess* fatigue as more severe soreness or pain, muscle imbalance producing a joint that hurts, or the inability to properly recover.

The real feeling of muscle fatigue may come from various levels of pain more than any other single sensation or movement. The brain interprets pain in an area called the limbic system—the emotional center. The idea of pain as an emotion is not new, and the symptom of excess fatigue is usually quite real. Our awareness of the problem in the brain allows our neurons to compensate for normal fatigue by improving fitness, or excessive fatigue by correcting related problems.

The brain can also teach our sometimes-stubborn conscious mind to avoid unhealthy training and racing, take adequate time to recover, and other healthy habits that help build fitness. This is referred to as intuition or instinct.

In a race, the brain uses the feeling of fatigue as a key regulator to insure that the event is completed as fast and successfully as possible, and without excessively damaging the body.

Dr. Timothy Noakes, in his writings about the importance of the athletic brain, states that, "the ultimate control of exercise performance resides in the brain's ability to vary the work rate and metabolic demand by altering the number of skeletal muscle motor units recruited during exercise." For many years, Noakes has discussed the physiological and emotional mechanisms, both unconscious and conscious, of muscle fatigue.

Fatigue and the Neuromuscular Mechanism

Every step you take starts with the brain sending messages to specific muscle fibers throughout the body to either contract or relax. In turn, and almost immediately, messages from each muscle fiber are sent to the brain with information about its status. In addition to the creation of physical movement and other aerobic benefits, this mechanism increases the brain's blood circulation (bringing in oxygen and other nutrients), stimulates the growth of new neurons (brain cells), and improves communication between cells. New neurological pathways between the brain and body are produced. The result is that you can build a better brain that takes care of your athletic body more effectively. And it does not take much: just a slow jog with proper warm up and cool down can do this, and actually increase the size of the brain by increasing the number of working brain cells and their interconnections (along with increased blood flow/circulation).

In addition to making movements more efficient, including improved balance and a better gait, the brain can benefit in more amazing ways. These include improvement of those areas associated with memory, cognition, social function, speech, hearing, behavior, and learning.

In order to train the full spectrum of aerobic muscle fibers, and its counterpart in the brain, an effective warm up and cool down is vital. This might mean spending a bit of time walking at the onset of a workout, and at the very end of it, to stimulate those muscles that move the body easily—otherwise, the full spectrum of aerobic fibers may not be trained. I recommend this routine regardless of the level of one's fitness.

It also means being serious and disciplined—and honest—about following a heart rate that helps keep the workout truly aerobic. In addition, rather than guessing your aerobic system is being properly trained, the MAF Test is an important monthly evaluation that more objectively measures these changes (see Appendix B).

It does not take long for these changes in the brain to occur—in fact, they begin during your very first high quality workout. And as the months pass the many physical changes that occur in the brain—and they can be significant—continue with each training session.

Performance and the brain

Effective racing involves pacing. I don't mean the mental strategy that involves our competitors, but rather, how the brain budgets muscle energy in our own body on a moment-to-moment basis. This helps create the ideal performance.

The sum total of all our physical experiences is recorded in the brain—a mechanism referred to as muscle memory. So not just any workout will do. Efficient training helps build a better brain leading to optimal performance. One of the best lessons about the athlete's brain can be found in a quote by Green Bay Packers' legendary coach Vince Lombardi: "Practice does not make perfect. Only perfect practice makes perfect." Optimal training is perfect practice, and it teaches the brain how best to perform.

Performance is a combination of many factors, which when not working well can cause excess muscle fatigue. Only when muscle fatigue is managed well can performance improve consistently and for a longer time. Training, nutrition, and stress are three key lifestyle factors that could either help the brain effectively manage fatigue, or not. Let's look at each topic.

- Training is obviously a key factor for optimal performance, and is associated with how the muscles are treated during physical activity. Minimizing fatigue is important, whether we are training for endurance, or strengthening bones and muscles. Yet, without stressing the body sufficiently, no training effect will occur. It is a question of balancing the quality of the workout or race, and the ability to recover from it. My traditional training equation is one that athletes should post in a prominent place where it can be seen every day: *Training = workout + recovery.*

  By far the most common mistake by athletes is too much training (intensity and-or duration), too little recovery (rest), or both. This results in excess muscle fatigue and brain function that is below par.

- Nutrition is another key factor for optimal muscle, brain, and race performance. This means eating the optimal diet for your needs. It starts by avoiding all junk food, including refined carbohydrates, fast food, and other harmful items.

  Muscles are continuously replacing old parts, so to speak, especially between workouts as part of the repair and recovery process. The building materials needed for these activities come from our diet. Along with all the vitamins and minerals, protein is particularly important to improve training and racing tolerance in muscles.

  Oxidative stress is associated with muscle fatigue, both at rest, and during physical activity. The aerobic muscle fibers utilize anti-oxidant nutrients for optimal function, including prevention of excess fatigue. Essentially, almost any nutrient is important for our anti-oxidant system, not just vitamins C and E, and others touted in ads. The best source of these substances is a healthy diet that includes 10 servings of fresh vegetables and fruits. Some of the more powerful foods include blueberries, blackberries, apples, beets, spinach, and kale. However, supplements of antioxidants may not only be ineffective, but also can worsen oxidative stress.

  Healthy fats are important too. In addition to the brain being 60 percent fat, this macronutrient regulates the body's inflammatory mechanisms, which can dramatically increase muscle fatigue.

Another factor associated with muscle fatigue is the increased levels of the brain's neurotransmitter *serotonin*. This chemical rises with the intake of high carbohydrate foods, and is reduced with the consumption of more complete protein.

- Stress regulation is another key aspect for great performance in the brain and body. It's simple: too much stress can increase muscle fatigue. The most obvious example is overtraining, which leads to poor muscle recovery, excess fatigue, and reduced performance.

Stress can be external from factors such as a bad job or relationship, overtraining, or poor diet; or internal from blood sugar impairments, mental or emotional strain, or poor training and racing strategies. In all stress situations, it's the brain that must deal with it. When successful, stress won't defeat us. But if not, our brain sends messages to the pituitary gland, and the adrenal glands, to try adapting. Muscle fatigue and other impairments, electrolyte imbalance (sodium deficiency), poor water regulation, and other problems result. In particular, the rise in the stress hormone cortisol reduces other hormones such as testosterone, which increases muscle fatigue. (Long training session greater than two hours can also reduce testosterone levels.)

With balanced training, diet, and stress control, increased aerobic function, and a better brain, muscle fatigue is significantly reduced and performance improves.

A checklist to help avoid this common problem:
One of the first truths we learn when studying the human body is that the brain controls virtually everything. In addition to managing the physical, chemical, and mental state, the brain has a mind of its own making each of us unique individuals. By taking care of the brain we can better manage muscle fatigue, and train and race up to our potential. Below are three key factors that can dramatically help the brain accomplish this task.

- *Health.* Overall, being a healthy athlete may be most important. When the body is functioning optimally, we reach our athletic potential more easily. All areas of health impact our fitness. It's simple. Healthier athletes are generally less injured, perform better, and don't have excess muscle fatigue. This is something we control to a great extent through better diet, reduced stress, and balanced training. A variety of brain-related features—mental, emotion, and psychological—can also influence muscle fatigue through the effects on perception, and on physiological variables such as heart rate, oxygen, and circulation. Those who are depressed, anxious, moody, or mentally stressed will not fare as well with fatigue compared to others.

    The sun has untold health benefits too. Sunlight stimulates the brain when the eyes are not covered by lenses or light blocked by windows. On the skin, sunlight can promote the production of vitamin D, which can directly reduce muscle dysfunction and fatigue.

- *Neuromuscular Factors.* The health of our muscles and the nerves controlling them are obviously important in preventing fatigue. This involves stimulating the neuromuscular system during workouts. Essentially, we "train" all the nerves and muscles in preparation for racing. This may seem obvious, but too many training routines don't adequately accomplish this. Stimulating the full spectrum of the aerobic muscle fibers is most important, and best accomplished by starting a workout slowly. This enlists those important fibers that move the body at a very low level of intensity, and perform important metabolic activities such as burning fat. A gradual increase in speed ultimately incorporates the full spectrum of movement from slow to moderately fast while maintaining sub-max training levels.

    Anaerobic fibers require training too, although much less as they are our "fight-flight" responders. Even the most untrained person can dash out of a sudden rainstorm or whisk across a busy city street. Most athletes also have at least one race in brain-muscle memory, and can easily turn this on while racing. In addition, endurance events rely almost exclusively on the aerobic system for energy needs, with a de-emphasis on the anaerobic system. These are some reasons why six months of aerobic-only training, for example, can result in a faster, personal-best race.

- *Gait.* By regulating the balance of muscle contraction and relaxation, the neuromuscular system plays a key role in creating a great gait. When this does not happen, the increase in muscle fatigue causes a poor gait. Generally, looking at the middle and back of the pack finishers of an endurance race shows more irregularity in movement than those finishing up front. When an athlete's gait is impaired, it costs more energy to cover each mile, impairing performance. Muscle fatigue itself will cause gait irregularity, so the problems of fatigue and poor gait perpetuate themselves (and usually include muscle imbalances). The cycle can often be broken by improved health and aerobic fitness. In stubborn cases, help from a healthcare professional may be necessary.

The above three factors are particularly important during a race. The brain works with the body we develop in training, and relies on the sum of all our nutrition, emotions, experiences, and every other aspect of health. If one part of the body functions less than optimal, the brain will be limited in how much it will ask of the body. For example, if our nutritional state is poor, muscle energy may be limited during a race. The brain will not allow an athlete to run faster than his ability and will slow the pace to protect the body. Likewise for muscle imbalance—rather than risk more serious injury, the brain will reduce performance to a level that is less harmful.

The brain subconsciously monitors and manages all the factors important for optimal muscle function, from oxygen and lactate to nutrient levels and ATP, and more. We can participate in this process by training with a heart monitor. This is a conscious form of biofeedback that can assist in building aerobic function and overall health, and help better understand the brain.

The Muscle Fatigue Checklist

Below is a checklist containing important items necessary for avoiding excess muscle fatigue. Make sure you're addressing all of them.

- Proper warm up—15 minutes for shorter training, 20 to 30 minutes for workouts lasting more than 90 minutes total.
- Proper cool down—just the opposite of warming up.
- Monitor the heart rate to help ensure the full spectrum of muscle fibers are trained.
- Each workout is without excess muscle fatigue or pain.
- Frequent rest (no training) or regular easy/short training days should be part of one's schedule.
- Adequate sleep: 7 to 9 hours uninterrupted each night.
- Wake up feeling rested and without physical discomfort.
- No depression, anxiety, moodiness, or other excess mental-emotional stress.
- Motivation for training and racing is high.
- Regular sun exposure on unprotected skin (without burning) and eyes (without glare).
- Feel good or great after training.
- Training, racing, and all other footwear is relatively flat and completely comfortable.
- Spend some time each day being barefoot.
- Increasing power or pace at same heart rate over time.
- Races end with energy for a finishing kick—you should have one each time!

These items are also factors that can help athletes improve health and significantly perform better.

Muscle Testing: Who, What, Where, and Why

Muscle testing is a procedure performed by health practitioners as part of a physical evaluation. It helps assess the body's muscles and their connections to the brain through the nervous system. Testing is accomplished by applying moderate and precise force against an arm, leg, or other body area of a patient who is simultaneously resisting in the opposite direction. This evaluation is particularly important for those with back, knee, and hip pain, spinal problems, wrist and elbow dysfunction, headaches, and many other disorders. Along with other evaluations, muscle testing can help practitioners determine the best therapy for their particular problems.

Testing muscles is a primary and practical way to determine a condition called muscle imbalance, where two or more muscles are not properly working together. The combination of a "tight," overactive muscle and one that is "loose" or less active is a simple but accurate definition of muscle imbalance. Because it is a common cause of injury, pain, and disability, the use of muscle testing can be as important as blood and urine evaluations, X-rays, physical examinations, and other assessments.

While associated with joint, ligament, tendon, and bone problems, muscle imbalance can significantly impair physical movement such as walking, reduce sports performance, and even lower the overall quality of life.

The Who

Muscle testing is used by a wide variety of practitioners, including those in medicine, osteopathy, chiropractic, physical therapy, and numerous others. For example, neurologists may perform it to help rule out serious conditions; physical therapists to rate a patient's level of disability; athletic trainers to assess a particular injury; and chiropractors to help determine areas of treatment. Overall, practitioners who employ biofeedback, manipulation, diet and nutrition, exercise, sports, coaching, and other approaches, often utilize muscle testing.

In the 1940s, physical therapists Florence and Henry Kendall developed a comprehensive system of manually testing muscles to evaluate disabilities. Their first textbook on the subject was published later that decade, and would inspire the work of two doctors, in uniquely different ways, and trigger a muscle testing revolution that continues today.

In the early 1960s, Vladimir Janda (1923–2002), a Czechoslovakian medical doctor, developed a system of care using muscle testing, teaching practitioners in many disciplines including physical therapists, athletic trainers, and chiropractors. Janda's primary approach included various therapies directed at the "tight" muscle, although sometimes he addressed the "loose" one to correct muscle imbalances.

Independently, and about the same time, George Goodheart (1918–2008), an American chiropractic physician, discovered a way to use muscle testing to evaluate the nervous system. In this approach, now used by chiropractors, medical doctors, osteopaths, and others, treatment incorporates a variety of complementary remedies including acupuncture, manipulation, and nutrition. Goodheart primarily directed therapy at the "loose" muscle (sometimes referred to as "weak"), and on occasion, applied treatment to the "tight" one to correct muscle imbalance.

The What

A term commonly associated with muscle testing is kinesiology, referring to the study of human movement. It is a topic taught in the coursework of many colleges and universities, and postdoctoral programs. Through an understanding of kinesiology, practitioners can better use muscle testing to evaluate posture, gait, and all other movements. Many types of assessment and treatment approaches incorporating muscle testing and using the name kinesiology have evolved over the last fifty years. Most originated from the work of Goodheart.

The Where

Tens of thousands of health practitioners around the world, in hospitals, clinics, private practice, on sports teams, and elsewhere, employ some form of muscle testing in their work. In addition, hundreds of studies have been published in scientific journals on this topic.

The Why

As an important part of a comprehensive physical evaluation, muscle testing can help discover the cause of a particular injury or disability. It can also quickly assist in measuring the effectiveness of specific treatments. While its use varies with individual practitioners, there is one common feature among all using it: muscle testing is a form of biofeedback.

We usually think of biofeedback as a type of electronic monitoring, such as EMG for muscles or EEG for the brain, which involves the use of electrical devices. While these approaches often incorporate muscle testing, most practitioners perform it as a hands-on evaluation without equipment. While millions of people have experienced muscle testing, many more have not. Finding a health practitioner who incorporates this form of evaluation is as easy as inquiring about whether testing muscles is part of his or her practice.

Muscles obviously play a key role in all sports, along with their energy requirement, blood that circulates through them, the nerves that stimulate them, and many other factors controlled by the brain. But when muscles are overused, they fatigue excessively, which can significantly impair training and performance. By limiting muscle fatigue to acceptable mild and moderate levels, optimal health and fitness can be better maintained.

EATING FOR ENDURANCE—ONE RULE FITS ALL

I have not abandoned my philosophy that we're all unique individuals. In fact, the idea is something referred to frequently in my articles, books, lectures and interviews. So what is this one rule that fits all? It's simple: avoid junk food. No one should eat it. I'm referring to our daily eating habits of meals, snacks, and desserts. There are always healthy alternatives—once junk food is gone your diet will fill up with real food.

I am not referring to the use of glucose and other carbohydrate nutrients important during long competitive events—an issue I've addressed in detail elsewhere.

One problem with junk food is that many people don't really know what it is because the world has been fed a lie for such a long time. The idea behind misguided marketing messages is easy—keep hitting people over the head with the same ridiculous idea and eventually they think it's very sensible, even necessary. Such is the case with junk food. Generations of people have been hearing the same foolish information—some of it even coming from governments, so-called health professionals, and others deemed "experts" in nutrition. As I've previously written, this is all in the name of money and politics, not health.

The fact is junk food is bad for physical, chemical, and mental health, and it can impair fitness. Let me explain the most important issue first.

What is Junk Food?

If you have to ask, you're probably eating it. Even small amounts are harmful—no, not just emotionally, but physiologically. And as most already know, junk food is a primary cause of the worldwide overfat epidemic that's affecting the full spectrum of individuals, from the poor to the most serious athletes.

In addition to its contribution to increased body fat, junk food may be the number one cause of the most common diseases, including cancer, diabetes, Alzheimer's, and heart disease, not to mention the problems that significantly contribute to low quality of life such as intestinal conditions, hormone imbalance, chronic inflammation, fatigue, and much more—even hair loss. For this reason, some health authorities want to refer to junk food as pathogenic food. But that won't happen soon enough thanks to the ongoing mult-million-dollar marketing campaigns waged by the food industry—the image of these bad foods is now being portrayed as harmless rather than the poison it really is.

However, pathologic food actually refers to its capability to cause pathological conditions, including those with excess body fat.

In all its many disguises—it's amazing how easy it is to fool even the very careful consumer—junk food, including soda, chips, candy, has resulted in one of the world's most successful business ventures. Large amounts of it are in almost all Western households, and in the East as well, including China, Japan, and Southeast Asia. It's even widespread in the Third World, where, in only a single generation, millions of starving people have now become overfat, thanks to junk food.

It's widely believed that the phrase *junk food* was coined in 1972 by Michael Jacobson, director of the American Center for Science in the Public Interest (a consumer advocacy organization that focuses on health and nutrition). But defining junk food has been a difficult task, partly because the numbers of items are alarmingly high, and also because the food landscape is always changing with new and improved products coming and going almost daily.

In defining junk food, the worst ones are most obvious—chips and cookies, colas and other sugared liquids, candy, and most other snacks. The biggest offenders are sugar (including sucrose, white table sugar, and others such as high fructose corn syrups and many others listed in Section 2) and flour, and the thousands of products made from these two deadly ingredients (from ketchup and mayonnaise to energy bars and sports products, and almost all liquid refreshments).

For those on the go, junk food is synonymous with fast food, and includes almost all burgers, fries, pizza, fried chicken, and foods that are battered or coated or have sauces. Included are the popular "salads," such as tuna and chicken salad, and even those low-cal dressings. Most international foods are not exempt from the junk-food category: Chinese food (high in sugar, starch, and-or flour), sushi (white rice with added sugar), sweetened teriyaki foods, deep fried fish and chips, and others.

Going to a deli for lunch? The popular ham and American cheese on a roll is entirely junk food. As is that pasta salad with crackers (almost all pasta, noodles, and similar items are junk). Of course, a plain bagel and Diet Coke is all junk food, too. Instead, have some leaf lettuce with tomatoes, red peppers, carrots, and slices of real roast beef or Swiss cheese. Hold the mayo and ketchup, but mustard (after reading the ingredients) or olive oil and vinegar would be OK.

As you push a shopping cart down the food store aisle, it's almost guaranteed that if the food is in a can, frozen, or wrapped in a package, it's probably junk food. Consider a can of peaches, which may seem healthy—but most are packed with high amounts of sugar. Instead, buy fresh fruit in season. Even most trendy bulk foods found in health stores and other retailers, with their funky image of pure and natural, is junk food.

Not only conventional foods available to consumers everywhere, but also most organic items found in health stores are junk, too. In fact, organic junk food is one of the fastest growing segments of the natural foods industry.

It's simple—there are two kinds of foods:

- *Healthy food.* It's real, naturally occurring, unadulterated and unprocessed, and nutrient-rich. If you can grow or raise it, it's real. Included are fresh fruits and vegetables, lentils and beans, eggs, real cheese, whole pieces of meat (such as fish, beef, chicken), nuts, seeds, and similar items. Consuming these foods provides a great potential for both immediate and long-term health benefits, with athletes reaping many benefits.
- *Junk food* is everything else. It's deceptively inexpensive to buy and unhealthy to eat. These items are processed, manufactured, have added chemicals, sugars, and other unhealthy ingredients that can immediately, and over the long term, adversely affect health and fitness. Unhealthy versions of healthy foods noted above include canned fruit in sugar-syrup, processed vegetables (canned, frozen, or from fast food outlets) with sugar, flour or chemicals, baked beans in a sugar and flour sauce, powdered and processed eggs with trans fats, processed cheese and cheese spreads, cold cuts (bologna, salami, chicken, and turkey loaf, fish sticks), peanut butter (typically containing sugar and trans fat), and roasted nuts (often with ingredients you can't even pronounce). Of course, genetically altered items, which are not allowed in certified organic foods or in many countries of the world, would also be considered junk food.

Can we rely on governments to help us understand what foods are junk and unhealthy? Not as long as the political influence by junk food lobbyists continues. This has resulted in some absurd ideas about food. For example, the United States Department of Agriculture (USDA), the federal department responsible for developing and executing U.S. food policies, does not consider a Snickers Bar to be junk food. How about chocolate chip cookies, high in white flour and sugar? Not junk food, says the USDA. Likewise for French fries, or the American version, and even an ice cream bar containing 320 calories with 4 teaspoons of sugar.

The USDA won't even address the food quality of school lunches. Their standards for foods and snacks sold out of vending machines, in cafeterias, and other venues only limit the sale of "foods of minimal nutritional value." The junk food industry gets around this issue by adding synthetic vitamins to their products and claim it's nutritious. One problem is that the USDA, which does not address calories, glycemic index, or the many hidden sugars, developed its standards in the 1970s, when most of today's junk food and knowledge of its health dangers—and marketing tricks—didn't exist.

Most people, including many junk food addicts, would agree that candy bars, cup cakes, colas, and similar hardcore unhealthy items are examples of classic junk foods. While this is true, there's a seemingly endless list of foods that many might not realize are unhealthy, with the same or very similar nutritional composition. These include almost all breakfast cereals, snack foods, breads, and packaged/prepared foods.

How much junk food causes harm? One bite can be enough for some people, especially those addicted to sugar. Certainly a junk food snack or meal can significantly alter one's physiology in a negative way. This seemingly small amount of junk can also switch on genes that trigger cancer, heart disease, Alzheimer's, obesity, and other common, preventable conditions.

Among the ways junk-food corporations make their products appear healthy, in addition to advertising, is through the fortification of processed flour. Virtually all this flour is used in prepared and packaged foods, including most baked goods, and what consumers buy for home cooking. In the processing of wheat flour, most vitamins are removed and lost. Food fortification, which exists in over 50 countries around the world, mandates that synthetic vitamins be added to processed flour.

There are at least two problems with this: first, it gives companies a way to advertise a junk food product as healthy ("contains 18 vitamins" or "100 percent of the daily need for folic acid"). Second, the policy of adding synthetic vitamins to one of the most commonly consumed foods in the world—white flour—has scientists concerned. Fortification has been halted in some countries due to, among other things, increased cancer rates from high intakes of folic acid.

Of course, vitamins are not the only nutrients removed from processed flour. Others include healthy fats, minerals, fiber and many phytonutrients. And, the great deception of "whole grain" is advertised everywhere—especially on packages of highly processed cereals, crackers, and other junk food.

The only truly whole grains that are not junk food are the real thing, wholesome kernels of oats, rice, wheat, rye, and others. Of course, most consumers have never seen wheat berries or the raw grains that occur in nature. You know they're real because they are whole pieces of real food that take much longer to cook. For example, oats in this form take 45 minutes or more to prepare. Compare this to junk food oats, which may take one minute to cook, or less as some oatmeal products only require that you add hot water.

Will governments finally encourage people to reduce or eliminate junk food? I would hope so. For one reason, no country can afford the overfat epidemic and its associated long list of chronic diseases, and with the reduction of the availability of unhealthy food, a dramatic drop in chronic disease would quickly follow. Not to mention raising quality of life everywhere.

But governments probably will not take this kind of action. Instead, they will rely on taxes. Cost, rather than intelligence or self-responsibility, is widely acknowledged by public health experts to have been the single biggest factor in reducing smoking rates. The same has started to happen with junk food. So far, New York City bans trans fats, Denmark became the first nation in the world to tax sugar, Romania has a new lower value-added tax rate on healthy foods, New Zealand is preparing to raise taxes on foods with little or no nutritional value, and other federal and regional governments are following suit. In addition, in various locations around the world there has been an increase in policies that restrict or ban junk foods in schools, and the same for television advertising during children's shows. (But even in schools where some unhealthy foods are banned, school lunches themselves consist of significant amounts of junk food.)

There is so much junk food in the world, and deception about it, that discussing it thoroughly could fill one or more books. Without junk food there are still plenty of delicious snacks, meals, and desserts.

As I've emphasized many times, eating well means planning ahead and carefully shopping so you always have only healthy food at home and work and during travel. By avoiding junk food I guarantee you'll quickly feel better, be healthier, and improve your overall human performance.

Beyond the Two-Week Test

The Two-Week Test is one of the more popular topics on my website (philmaffetone.com). This dietary self-evaluation has been used by untold numbers of people, most of whom felt and performed better, lost weight, and improved fat burning. If you have not read about this test, you can also see either of the Big books listed in the Preface.

Many people have asked me how I developed the Two-Week Test. That story should also be part of understanding the Test, so I describe it here.

I developed the Two-Week Test in the mid-1980s. After spending almost seven years trying to wean carbohydrate-intolerant patients off white flour and sugar, it was exhausting work—almost like dealing with drug addicts. My goal was to lower carbohydrate intake to find the level that would eliminate signs and symptoms of excess insulin. The process went too slowly.

One evening I was reading the *Merck Manual*, the most popular medical reference book used by many healthcare professionals to look up basic facts about assessment and treatment procedures. There was a single sentence, almost an aside, about elevations of insulin and how reducing carbohydrates might be necessary in some patients with *hyperinsulinemia* (too much insulin).

Then I recalled a 1971 study from the *New England Journal of Medicine*. It was tucked away with copies of other studies in a folder called "Blood Sugar and Insulin" in my filing cabinet. As I paged through the study called "Effect of Diet Composition on the Hyperinsulinemia of Obesity" the proverbial pieces to the puzzle starting falling into place. Then I recalled another study. I searched the file hoping to find it. There it was, from Columbia University's Department of Medicine and published in the *Journal of Clinical Investigation* in 1976 ("Composition of Weight Lost during Short-term Weight Reduction"). It showed that ten days of restricted carbohydrate foods resulted in not only the loss of weight, but also a reduction of body fat.

This information was not really new to me, it was the reason I was weaning patients' off insulin-provoking foods. But for some reason, the short excerpt, and the other two studies brought everything into clearer focus. I asked myself, "If weaning patients off their unhealthy carbohydrate addiction was so difficult, why not go 'cold turkey' so they could experience the immediate benefits? They would actually feel better quickly because insulin levels would drop right away, and within the first few days they would begin to experience life without harmful levels of this hormone rather than by slowly reducing those foods, which could take weeks or months to attain the same effect."

At first, this new test period I devised lasted ten days—the same period of time used in one of the studies I had reviewed. But the first few patients I used this new approach on needed more time off carbohydrates to fully appreciate the positive effects, particularly with regard to burning body fats. I added four more days to the trial or test period. Two weeks worked much better.

To be sure patients understood this was not a diet, I referred to it as a test. It eventually became known in my office as the Two-Week Test.

The Two-Week Test was unique. Not only because it helped me better understand the patient's sensitivity to carbohydrate foods; but more importantly, rather than conducting a blood or urine test that provided numbers that most patients could not easily understand or translate to real-life changes, this new approach required individuals to take an active role in the process of self-evaluation. During the testing period, he or she would actually feel what it was like to have normal insulin levels, optimal blood sugar and, in many cases, be finally free of signs and symptoms associated with CI—all within a short time frame. This was a far superior method of educating the patient.

For those individuals who were not carbohydrate intolerant and didn't feel any different during the test, it ruled out CI as a common health problem. However, this did not mean they could consume white sugar and other refined carbohydrates such as white flour—ingredients that were becoming the bulk of many diets. But patients who were overweight, had blood-sugar problems, and simply could not escape the damage of eating refined carbohydrates now knew what it would take to quickly change their health.

Going *beyond* the Two-Week Test means we can skip over the period of experimentation, and just avoid all junk food.

But there is still one reason to do the Test, or a version of it—because many people are unable to tolerate more than small amounts of *natural* carbohydrates. While we think of fresh fruit, honey, lentils, beans, and other natural foods as healthy, some don't tolerate that amount of carbohydrates each day. As discussed in Section 1, further lowering insulin levels, which could help increased fat burning even more and trigger the production of more ketone bodies (also used for energy), is necessary for some people.

Two more examples of the world's population being swindled into eating junk food follow. The nutrients discussed next are two that are commonly found in low levels in athletes.

Vitamin A and the Beta-Cartotene Myth

While we think of vitamin A as being described as something to prevent night blindness, this essential nutrient goes far beyond that notion, especially for athletes.

Vitamin A was first discovered in butterfat and cod liver oil in 1913. While these two foods are still great sources of this vital nutrient, fruits and vegetables don't have any of it. Many are surprised by this, and it's one reason millions of people don't get enough vitamin A. The result is reduced human performance, poor aging, and potential problems in virtually all areas of the body.

There are three key reasons why so many people don't get enough vitamin A.

- First, vitamin A is only found in animal foods. It's a myth that plant foods are full of this nutrient. Instead, fruits and vegetables are high in a family of phytonutrients called carotenoids. The body must convert three of these compounds—beta-carotene, alpha-carotene, and beta-cryptoxanthin—to vitamin A. But in humans, this conversion is quite inefficient, with about 10 to 20 molecules of carotenoids needed to make one of vitamin A. In addition, 80 percent or more of natural vitamin A from animal sources is absorbed, but only 3 percent or less of carotenoids from plant foods are absorbed.

- Second is that there are a number of genetic variants, mutations similar to those described for folate (discussed later in this section), which can significantly impair the body's ability to convert the carotenoids to vitamin A. This genetic problem may exist in up to half of the population. Its presence appears to be associated with high blood levels of beta-carotene, alpha-carotene, beta-cryptoxanthin, and low levels of lycopene, lutein, and zeaxanthin—three other carotenoids important for health but that don't convert to vitamin A.
- Third, in healthy individuals, vitamin A is continuously being used for many functions throughout the body as noted below. Most vitamin A is stored in the liver, and about 5 percent of it is used up each day, which must be replaced by sufficient dietary sources.

Because of these three important factors, we must get our vitamin A from animal sources to avoid the risk of low levels. The best sources are meats, including liver, beef, chicken, and turkey, dairy, especially cheese and butter, and egg yolks. It's obvious this means finding healthy, organic, or otherwise real foods. Likewise, dietary supplements of cod liver oil are the best.

Vitamin A Complex

Vitamin A is not a single nutrient but actually a complex group of compounds called retinoids, of which many forms exist in nature and in the body. Each form of vitamin A performs functions the others cannot. For example, retinol is the major transport and storage form of vitamin A; retinal is essential for vision, and retinoic acid has hormone actions and regulates more than five hundred genes.

In addition to the poor conversion of carotenoids to vitamin A, two important factors are also necessary for the body to obtain this vitamin from plant sources. Good gut function, especially stomach, gall bladder, liver, and small intestines, is necessary for optimal absorption. While vitamin A is found in foods containing fat, the carotenoids are often not, making the addition of fat in the meal important for their absorption.

Conversion of carotenoids takes place in the small intestines (with some in the liver and kidney), first to the retinol form of vitamin A. This process requires other nutrients including riboflavin, niacin, iron, zinc, and adequate dietary protein.

Labeling laws are allowed to maintain the myth that beta-carotene is the same as vitamin A. Read any label on a plant-based product and it lists the amount of vitamin A. Likewise for dietary supplements—most don't have any vitamin A even when labeled as such (except for those containing synthetic A, the most common source used in both fortification and supplementation). What the label really refers to is the vitamin A equivalent under ideal circumstances. For example, to obtain 1 mcg (microgram) of vitamin A as retinol it takes 10 mcg of beta-carotene, and 20 mcg of alpha-carotene or beta-cryptoxanthin. However, for labeling purposes, dietary supplements can claim that to obtain 1 mcg of vitamin A, 2 mcg of beta-carotene is required—the assumption is that the pill will be taken on an empty stomach with no other food taken with or soon after it, and digestion and absorption will be ideal.

Signs, symptoms, or increased risk of vitamin A insufficiency or deficiency are many. Below are 20 common ones. How many do you have?

1. Increased sun exposure
2. Reduced immunity
3. Recurrent infections, especially viral and fungal
4. Chronic intestinal problems
5. Liver dysfunction
6. Poor night vision
7. Female of childbearing age
8. Low fat diet

9. Vegetarian diet
10. Macular degeneration
11. Dry skin
12. Dry hair
13. Dry mucous membranes
14. Weak or ridged fingernails
15. Chronic inflammation
16. Allergies or asthma
17. Weak bones or teeth
18. Difficulty maintaining vitamin D levels
19. Excess body fat
20. History of cancer

In addition to acne, psoriasis, and a few conditions, much of the research around vitamin A is related to cancer. Studies show that eating foods rich in vitamin A, not carotenoids, is linked to a lower risk of cancer, while others demonstrate vitamin A can also prevent normal cells from becoming cancer. Others show this nutrient can slow tumor growth, shrink tumors, and make some cancer treatments work better.

The relationship between better brain function and vitamin A is also very important, with many clinicians using this nutrient in adults and children with a wide range of neurological deficits, including those with learning and memory problems.

The recommended daily allowance (RDA) of vitamin A is between 2,310 IU (0.7 milligrams) per day for adult women (more for women who are pregnant or breastfeeding), and 3,000 IU (0.9 milligrams) per day for men, with children needing less. (Vitamin A is still listed on food and supplement labels in international units—IUs—even though scientists rarely use this measure.)

Blood tests for vitamin A as retinol, and even for carotenoid levels, are typically measured in a simple blood test. However, the value of blood tests for assessing true vitamin A status is limited because this nutrient does not decline in the blood until vitamin A levels in the liver are almost depleted.

The best source of vitamin A is cod liver oil. But if you're taking a high dose of vitamin D (such as 5 to 10,000 IUs or more) take your dose of A in the morning and D in the evening (or the other way around) as vitamin D can reduce the absorption of vitamin A.

Low intakes of carotenoids are associated with poor health, in particular, chronic disease and disability, so continue eating your ten servings of fruits and vegetables—studies show consuming them is protective against the decline in physical performance, and overall mortality. But carotenoids and vitamin A are two separate groups of nutrients. And don't rely on beta-carotene or other phytonutrients to provide adequate vitamin A levels. Instead, get your vitamin A from animal foods, or supplements of cod liver oil.

The Folate Plot

Athletes need, among other things, a more than adequate amount of red blood cells to carry oxygen throughout the body. Making these cells requires the nutrient called folate.

The discovery in 1991 that about 70 percent of neural tube defects, a group of serious birth defects, could be prevented by the consumption of synthetic folic acid led to a major health promotion campaign in many Western countries, by governments, and those in healthcare and industry. The objective would be for women to take 400 micrograms (mcg) of synthetic folic acid daily before getting pregnant. Authors of a just published study (Andrew Boilson and colleagues in a 1996 issue of the *American Journal of Clinical Nutrition*) state that "This campaign largely failed in its objective, in part because more than half of all pregnancies are unplanned."

For decades before this time, synthetic folic acid was a part of most dietary supplements sold in drug and health stores, and in prescription forms. Often, they are sold as "natural" even though they are not.

By 1998, pharmaceutical companies, the manufacturers of synthetic folic acid, increased their business when governments mandated that processed flour be fortified with this chemical. As of 2007, fifty-two countries worldwide had national regulations mandating folic acid fortification. This strategy, along with the popular recommendation for women of childbearing age to take folic acid continued. Boilson and colleagues conclude that, "After twenty years, the risks and/or benefits associated with either of these strategies remains unclear, and the debate continues."

Part of the debate is that some scientists and health authorities are changing their mind. The United Kingdom suspended their fortification program when they discovered an increase in cancer rates attributable to the addition of folic acid. Ireland has just stopped its program as well.

Researchers also noticed that rates of colorectal cancer went up in North America around the same time that fortification began. They estimate that excess folic acid consumption may cause an additional fifteen thousand cases of colorectal cancer each year in the U.S. and Canada. By comparison, fortification prevents an estimated two to three thousand cases of neural tube defects in both countries.

Another study showed the same problem in Chile after fortification began there in 2000—increased rates of colorectal cancer.

The latest concern is an increased risk of prostate cancer. So it's not any one specific cancer, but quite possibly any form. Folic acid can speed up cancers for the same reason it can prevent neural tube defects—the body uses more folate for rapid cell growth, something shared in the fetus and tumors.

More than fifty years ago, research showed that synthetic folic acid supplements accelerated leukemia in children. (Such studies helped lead to a class of antifolate drugs that are among today's most common cancer treatments.)

In 1941, the food form of folate was first discovered in green leafy vegetables (folate from the Latin word for leaf, *folium*). Since then, hundreds of studies have shown the benefits of naturally occurring folate, while none show any harm.

But recent studies have been demonstrating the potential ill effects of long-term synthetic folic acid intake. Part of the problem is that too many people are getting too much because so many processed foods are fortified with this chemical. In fact, current levels of synthetic folic acid are in excess by as much as twice the target set for fortification.

When reading the ingredient list on a food package, if it states "folic acid," it's the synthetic version.

I refer to the chemical as "synthetic" because it does not exist in natural even in any modest amounts, and it has to be changed when humans consume it to an active form of folate—the same ones that exist in natural food. This issue is further discussed later.

There have always been safety issues surrounding the use of this synthetic vitamin. In addition to the prevalence of leukemia, another concern was related to the masking effect of folic acid on vitamin B12 deficiency, the cause of pernicious anemia. The lack of adequate B12 can come from poor diet (not consuming animal foods) or poor absorption from the intestines (due to stress or disease). This form of anemia can occur at any age, although symptoms don't usually appear until after age thirty, there is a higher prevalence in those over sixty.

Untreated pernicious anemia can produce little or no symptoms in many patients. In others it can cause fatigue, shortness of breath, poor concentration, and depression. It can also be fatal in some cases. That's because this form of anemia can severely affect the brain.

It's not likely that the U.S. will suspend fortification of processed foods with synthetic folic acid any time soon. The business of selling these and other synthetic vitamins, whether for fortification or pills, is booming.

Xinfa Pharmaceuticals, a Chinese manufacturer of folic acid, produces in excess of 1,200 tons per year, with probably most finding its way to U.S. retail shelves. Turned into tablets, that amount of folic acid can produce more than four trillion pills. I don't have data on how much of this folic acid goes to the fortification program. But the dietary supplement industry in the U.S. is a multi-billion dollar business alone. As is well known, the pharmaceutical industry has thousands of lobbyists in Washington, DC, who try to influence Congress. The non-partisan *Center for Public Integrity* reported that the pharmaceutical industry spent $855 million on lobbying activities between 1998 and 2006.

The primary problem is nothing more than the fact that too many people are not eating well. Governments have not helped, allowing—actually encouraging—industry to sweet-talk entire populations into avoiding the consumption of healthy food by offering easy, cheap, and unhealthy alternatives. Typical government and health care recommendations are to consume large amount of carbohydrates, which usually means people eat a lot of refined flour that's fortified with synthetic vitamins. By not eating fresh fruits and vegetables, for example, the primary sources of adequate natural folates, along with legumes, millions of people are choosing junk food instead, void of essential natural nutrients.

Folate Versus Folic Acid

It's important to differentiate between natural folates in foods, and synthetic folic acid in vitamin pills and fortified processed foods. By convention, the term "folic acid" refers specifically to the synthetic form of the vitamin. Chemically, it's fully oxidized, a non-coenzyme, and inactive because it can't be used in this form by the body. This compound is used in dietary supplements and fortified foods, because it's cheap and very stable.

In nature, there is a family of folates naturally occurring in various foods. Like other natural vitamins, they are biologically active as coenzymes in the body, helping many vital reactions in the prevention of disease.

Cancer is one of the conditions that natural folates help prevent, as studies have long shown. But because folate helps the body regulate a substance called homocysteine, it can also significantly reduce the risk of cardiovascular disease. While studies show that dietary folate reduces the risk of cardiovascular disease, the same cannot be said of synthetic folic acid. In an evaluation of previous studies, Lydia Bazzano and colleagues at Tulane University School of Public Health concluded that, "Folic acid supplementation has not been shown to reduce risk of cardiovascular diseases."

In addition, depression and other brain disorders including cognitive dysfunction such as Alzheimer's disease can be prevented and treated by natural folates. However, with few exceptions, dietary supplements of synthetic folic acid have not been shown to accomplish these feats.

Once inside the body, all forms of this vitamin—the food folates and folic acid—are converted to the most metabolically active folate called 5-methyltetrahydrofolate or 5-MTHF. The intestines and liver play the key roles in enabling this process. Recent studies show that the liver is limited in its ability to metabolize folic acid in oral doses greater than 260 to 280 mcg. Amounts beyond this can overwhelm the body's metabolism, according to researchers, resulting in unmetabolized folic acid, or UFA.

Potential Problems of UFA

In the case of folic acid, if conversion to 5-MTHF does not occur effectively, which can take place when too much of the synthetic form is consumed, UFA can accumulate in the blood. While this may be a marker that excess synthetic and or fortified foods have been consumed, UFA is associated with a variety of potential health problems. These include:

- Impairment of the body's production of natural killer cells weakening the immune system. Natural killer cells are an important part of our body's immune response, capable of killing tumor cells and viruses, for example. (It's now known that natural folate can also act as a powerful antioxidant.)

- High folic acid intake may increase the risk of cognitive decline with aging. A recent study at Tufts University showed a relationship between UFA and lower cognitive test scores in subjects 60 years and older. This study also showed that those consuming alcoholic beverages combined with circulating UFA can interact synergistically to precipitate anemia even in the absence of vitamin B12 deficiency. This translates to nearly two million elderly who might be at increased risk of cognitive impairment.
- Individuals who have detectable levels of unmetabolized folic acid may represent a subpopulation that has altered folic acid metabolism. This may be associated with specific genetic defects.
- In pregnant women, high folic acid in the blood may increase the risk of insulin resistance and obesity in their children.
- Synthetic folic acid may actually reduce the body's ability to metabolize food folates, and prevent the conversion of folic acid to its most active form, 5-MTHF.

Unfortunately, many people are unable to convert folic acid to the natural active form due to a genetic disorder, a problem that could further increase UFA.

What You Can Do

Eating sufficient amounts of foods to provide adequate folate is important for everyone. This means consuming real food and avoiding junk food. This is accomplished when enough vegetables are consumed, the best sources of folate, along with other items including fruits, legumes, and meats (even cocoa has a moderate amount). The chart below lists some of these folate-rich foods.

SOME FOLATE-RICH FOODS

FOOD (single serving)	Folate (mcg)
Avocado	118
Spinach	263
Asparagus	243
Beets	136
Leaf lettuce	119
Lentils	358
Brussels sprouts	157
Broccoli	168
Green peas	94
Orange	54
Papaya	112
Turkey	486
Beef	221

Source: USDA database.

These are not the only foods high in natural folates, so variety is important—beans, broccoli, Brussels sprouts, chicken, and many other items also contain significant levels of folate.

Loss of water-soluble folate during cooking is not significant unless foods are boiled in water and the water discarded. Steaming, grilling, baking, sautéing, and other forms of cooking are acceptable. However, raw vegetables in particular need to be chewed well in order to obtain the folate within these foods. For this reason, blending is most effective in obtaining high amount of food folate. An example is the addition of raw spinach to your smoothie (you won't even know it's there with a little sweetness from fresh fruits).

Genetic variants that impair human performance and cause disease.

A key benefit to obtaining folate in natural foods, which directly affects our overall health and fitness, is that this nutrient is required for a biochemical process called methylation.

Methylation is essential for the proper function of almost all the body's systems. It occurs billions of times every second, playing a key role in:

- Repairing DNA damage
- Detoxification
- Brain function
- Controlling inflammation
- Controlling which genes are turned on or off (such as those for cancer, diabetes, heart disease, and Alzheimer's)

Inadequate folate levels increase the risk for many health problems. These include a variety of cancers, osteoporosis, diabetes, Alzheimer's and other dementias, stroke and heart disease, neural tube defects, spontaneous abortion, male infertility, and possibly Down syndrome.

In the study noted above, which reported a 70 percent reduction in neural tube defects from folic acid supplementation, researchers speculated that mothers of the other 30 percent with these defects may not have been responsive to folic acid.

It appears that these women may be unable to convert synthetic folic acid to the active form of folate used in the body, 5-methyltetra-dydrofolate (5MTHF), due to a genetic variant.

This genetic problem is called the C677TT genotype, "T" variant, or polymorphism, and its occurrence is relatively new at such high levels in the population. It's particularly a common problem seen in difficult patients who appear unresponsive to many therapies.

What began as a mutation seen in very few individuals a generation ago is now common. (Each parent supplies genes to their child, and the polymorphism is passed on when one or both parents have the genetic variant in their chromosomes.)

Today, many millions of the world's population has the polymorphism, with geographic and ethnic variation. For example, U.S. Hispanics and Southern Europeans have frequencies above 40 percent, with other European populations (including British and Irish) and U.S. whites between 30 and 36 percent. Lower incidences are seen in U.S. black and Asian populations (14 and 11 percent, respectively).

How much does this polymorphism effect folate metabolism? Significantly. If two parents have the genetic variant, and pass both to the offspring, they are "homozygous" (meaning they received the variant from both parents), and their ability to convert folic acid to the natural folate (5MTHF) is reduced by 70 percent. Children who receive the variant from one parent have a 35 percent reduction. About half the general population carries at least one type of polymorphism.

Consequently, despite consuming enough folic acid from fortified food or synthetic dietary supplements, deficiency can commonly occur, even if blood levels of folic acid are normal. Knowing whether you, your partner, or your children have this polymorphism is accomplished with a simple blood test (discussed below).

The polymorphism has not only become common, but also its incidence is rising rapidly in some populations. The cause appears to be environmental.

Folate deficiency can cause chromosome breaks. Some researchers think that low dietary folate levels due to reduced vegetable and fruit intake adversely affected our genes giving rise to a genetic variant, which then impairs our ability to metabolize folic acid. This was one of the arguments that led to fortification of flour with synthetic folic acid.

However, it's also been theorized that the cause of so many polymorphisms today is high levels of unmetabolized folic acid (UFA) from high intakes of synthetic folic acid. In animal studies, higher levels of this vitamin can adversely affect DNA, and these changes influence subsequent generations. There is concern that the same problem is occurring in humans. In Spain, for example, the prevalence of the polymorphism has reportedly doubled since the introduction in 1982 of folic acid supplements for women in early pregnancy.

Those with the polymorphism may be particularly vulnerable to brain dysfunction. This is due to the inability of folic acid to get into the brain (it can't cross the blood-brain barrier), while natural folates can. In addition to the conditions noted above, this also places these individuals at increased risk for depression, mood and behavioral problems, schizophrenia, bipolar disorder, and other brain problems.

The polymorphism appears to also increase the risks of intestinal dysfunction, including Crohn's disease and ulcerative colitis. This is because natural folates play such crucial roles in various areas of the intestinal tract.

Folates are also vital in the regulation of red blood cells, and the polymorphism can lead to folate-deficient or megaloblastic anemia (where the cells are abnormally large). Since red blood cells carry oxygen, low folate can impair physical activity and be associated with fatigue. Symptoms may be more noticeable at higher altitudes, where oxygen uptake is already lower. In athletes it can significantly reduce performance.

The genetic polymorphism is also commonly associated with high levels of blood homocysteine, which is measured in a simple blood test. High homocysteine is associated with cardiovascular disease (along with recurrent embryo loss in early pregnancy and neural tube defects), and is a good measure of one's folate status.

Folic Acid Safety

It has now been years since researchers started questioning the use of fortification of folic acid at such high levels, and the possible genetic and disease consequences. According to the U.S. Institute of Medicine, a safe upper limit of folic acid intake is 1,000 mcg for adults and 300 to 800 for children, depending on age. However, there is no consensus about what blood concentrations of unmetabolized folic acid might cause harm (this form is due to the inability of the body to convert synthetic folic acid to a natural form). According to research, the upper limit of safety appears to be around 59 nmol/L.

Those with the highest blood concentrations of folic acid are children aged five years and under. While 43 percent of these children had blood concentrations approaching the limit of 50, 10 percent had levels above 77. This is astonishing, and reflects intake of junk food, high in fortified synthetic folic acid.

The intake of folic acid needed to achieve these blood levels has been estimated by researchers: 43 percent of children five years and older are consuming in excess of 780 mcg of synthetic folic acid each day. This is double the proposed tolerable upper limit (300–400 mcg) for children of that age. Even more alarming is that 10 percent are consuming over 1,320 mcg per day, which is well above the tolerable upper limit for adults. High levels were also found in children aged six to eleven years, and those over the age of sixty. The potential harm is a particular problem in children who are at a rapid stage of development when susceptibility to genetic damage is high. In addition, a mother's folate status can influence the child's genes.

Dietary Supplement Options

For those with higher folate needs, those who can't or won't eat sufficient amounts of healthy food, two types of dietary supplements are helpful.

- The body's most useful folate, 5MTHF, is available as a dietary supplement. This would be the best folate form to use for fortification, but that will never happen due to higher costs. This may be the most useful supplement for those with polymorphism.

Many nutrition-oriented health professionals use this nutrient, but it's more difficult to find in stores.

- Another form of folate, also available as a dietary supplement, is called folinic acid. It too converts to 5MTHF in the body but some folinic acid is used in different biochemical pathways, especially in the synthesis of DNA and regulation of genetic materials. Clinicians sometimes use folinic acid as a dietary supplement along with 5MTHF, for brain-related problems and other conditions. (Patients who take the drug metholtrexate, used to treat rheumatoid arthritis and various cancers, are often given high doses of folinic acid to recover the significant loss of folate from the drug's side effect. Many NSAIDs and other medications also have antifolate activities, reducing the body's level of folate.)

Blood Tests

Along with other assessments, blood tests may be very useful to help determine folate-related problems. Here are some tests your health practitioner may perform:

- Homocysteine. This is one of the most common and accurate measures of folate status.
- Genetic test for C677T. Three potential results are negative (normal), heterozygous (one variant), and homozygous (two variants).
- Red blood cell count (including indices). This measures the quantity and quality of the cells and helps rule out anemia.
- Unmetabolized folic acid (not performed by all laboratories).
- Fasting serum folate and erythrocyte folate. (Most laboratories don't differentiate between synthetic folic acid and 5MTHF.)

Many people have health problems associated with folate insufficiency or deficiency. The first factor in addressing these conditions is to assure sufficient amounts of natural folate from *food* are being consumed (see Part 1). In many cases, it's also important to know if the genetic polymorphism exists, and whether the body is using adequate amounts of folate as indicated by homocysteine levels. This information can easily be obtained from blood tests. The second consideration is supplementing the diet as necessary.

The Folate Survey

The survey below lists the most common indications of the increased need for natural folates. How many do you have?

1. History or risk of heart disease
2. History or risk of Alzheimer's disease or reduced mental capacity
3. Female of childbearing age
4. Outdoors often in sun or use tanning salons
5. Live in southern climates (below Washington DC)
6. Over age fifty
7. Chronic anemia
8. Feelings of depression
9. History of taking high doses of vitamin C (above 500 mg)
10. Reduced intake of meat, fish.
11. Eat less than two egg yolks per day.
12. Increased caffeine intake (coffee, tea, soda—more than three per day)
13. Increased alcohol intake (more than two drinks per day)
14. Cigarette smoking, or recent history.
15. Consume less than ten servings of fresh fruits and vegetables per day.

Even one or two of these indications may mean an increased need for folates. At the very least it means you should have your homocysteine levels measured with a blood test, or perform other evaluations as discussed in Section 2.

Many foods contain natural folates. Raw, fresh spinach, for example, may be one of the highest rated folate foods. Reductions in folates occur with food storage (folate breaks down over time), and during freezing, canning, and cooking. But if you're eating adequately, and still have high homocysteine, it may mean your folate is still low and you may require natural supplementation.

Nutrients That Support Folate

In addition to obtaining natural folates from a healthy diet, other nutrients help with their regulation. This is especially important for those individuals who are genetically compromised with the C677T genotype. For example, consumption of apples, especially the skins, can help the body compensate for genetic insufficiency, thereby preventing the adverse effects of such problems as low folate and high homocysteine. This is probably due to the fruits many phytonutrients, especially those with antioxidant functions.

The high antioxidant content of fruits and vegetables can impact our health many ways. One is that these nutrients can protect against gene disorders, including the C677T genotype. So eating more fruits and vegetables not only provides the vitamins and minerals necessary for good health, they protect us in other ways against genetic and other disorders, many of which are still not completely understood.

Those with the genetic variant may compensate to some degree for low folate status by utilizing more of the nutrient choline (which, like folate, can serve as a methyl donor) This includes helping to reduce abnormally high homocysteine levels. An increased need for choline is common, especially in those under higher levels of stress, and with asthma. The main dietary source of this nutrient is in egg yolks (with none found in the whites).

Based on the amount needed to prevent liver dysfunction, the government recommends only about 500 mg of choline for adults. But even this amount is very difficult to obtain from the diet without consuming eggs everyday—something the government recommends against.

More importantly, the metabolic requirement for choline is likely higher in individuals with the genetically compromised folate status. At the same time, choline also helps protect against genetic damage, which is the earliest functional effect of its inadequacy.

In addition, omega-3 fats from fish oil have been shown to positively influence genetic expression, and improve the function of the enzymes necessary to metabolize folates.

Two other nutrients important in folate metabolism include riboflavin (vitamin B2) and magnesium.

If this subject seems complicated, it is. These three relatively short articles don't do the topic justice. However, the remedy for these problems is very simple: eat your fruits and vegetables. And if you need additional folate, use a supplement containing natural forms of folate.

Chocolate Lovers Live Longer

Real cocoa can help your muscles move better, promote graceful aging, enhance brainpower, and reduce the risk of heart disease, cancer, and Alzheimer's—and it's healthy and fun to eat.

Off the northern coast of Panama in the south Caribbean Sea lie the San Blas Islands. For generations, the Kuna natives who live there have consumed large amounts of the fruits from the Malvaceae tree, an evergreen native to the tropics of the Americas. The fruits are also known as theobroma cacao, or cocoa as it's come to be known. Theobroma is from the Greek, meaning "food of the gods."

The Kuna, whose main beverage is made from cocoa, have great longevity and a very low incidence of many diseases. Harvard Medical School's Dr. Norman Hollenberg and colleagues studied the people living on the San Blas Islands, along with neighboring Panamanians who ate similarly but did not use much cocoa. The researchers found the non-cocoa consumers had more than a 1,000 percent higher incidence of heart disease, and a more than 600 percent increase in cancer.

Many studies have long shown that a group of phytonutrients called flavonoids (also referred to as bioflavonoids or flavanols) could help prevent cardiovascular disease, cancer and many other chronic illnesses. Cocoa is the richest natural food source of these nutrients. However, just grabbing a candy bar or instant hot chocolate won't give you many healthy benefits because processed cocoa—the most common form available—has a significantly reduced content of flavonoids. Most of these products also contain harmful, high-glycemic sugars, unhealthy dairy, and other ingredients that can actually contribute to illness.

Flavonoids exert powerful effects on blood vessels, one of the reasons they can reduce blood pressure and improve heart function. Those with blood sugar problems are particularly vulnerable to circulatory problems, and these individuals may especially benefit from cocoa's nutrition. There are, perhaps, more than a billion of these people on earth who are carbohydrate intolerance—probably 100 million in the U.S. alone. Their conditions include the full spectrum of diabetes, those with abnormal blood sugar regulation, and other problems with varying degrees that lead to blood vessel complications. When chronic, this circulatory distress can damage the liver, muscles, and the nervous system, including the brain. These individuals should avoid all refined carbohydrates, especially sugar, and make their own low-glycemic, healthy cocoa-rich foods.

Cocoa's phytonutrients include many other compounds, including the powerful group of polyphenols, but most research has focused on the health benefits of flavonoids. These include some very specific actions in the body. First is the increased natural production of nitric oxide, a compound that can significantly improve the function of blood vessels to increase circulation. This means more nutrient-rich blood is delivered to organs, glands, muscles, and bones, and more metabolic byproducts are removed.

In the case of the brain, consuming cocoa has been shown to improve circulation for two to three hours after consumption. This makes having a Phil's Bar or other cocoa snack a valuable asset before an important meeting, a long drive, or for students taking tests. But this idea can backfire if eating a high glycemic product, which can impair brain function.

Flavanol-rich cocoa may also work much like aspirin to promote better circulation by preventing blood platelets from sticking together.

In addition to improving circulation, flavonoids are powerful antioxidants. As such they can control chemicals called free radicals, which cause us to age quicker and increase the risk of many diseases.

The production of nitric oxide and antioxidant action can also improve muscle function. This is particularly important when working out, and especially for competitive athletes—and, need I say, for aging muscles, which are more easily damaged by free radicals.

Don't be fooled into thinking you can get all your antioxidants in a pill—you can't. Many studies in past decades have shown the vital need to obtain these key nutrients from foods, especially fresh fruits and vegetables, and cocoa; while other studies have failed to demonstrate dietary supplements containing antioxidants can accomplish the same.

With all these wonderful healthy nutrients from a food consumed by millions of people in large amounts, one might think the benefits would be more apparent, such as less heart disease, high blood pressure, and cancer. Just like there are two kinds of healthy desserts—chocolate and everything else—there are two very different types of chocolate: health and unhealthy.

Healthy vs. Unhealthy

Most people eat unhealthy chocolate contained in foods such as desserts, shakes, energy bars, and various types of candies. But it's all junk food, including the vast majority of products sold in health stores—even the organic versions. As such, these foods diminish health starting with the first bite. This is due to the many bad ingredients used to make these products, most notably white sugar, often disguised as cane juice, beet sugar, and other fancy names.

When making your own chocolate recipes, use only pure cocoa—without sugar, dairy, or other unwanted ingredients. While these forms of cocoa are not always easy to find (because junk food cocoa is cheaper and more readily available), healthy cocoa comes in powder and solid forms, as dark, unsweetened cocoa. Use these options to make your own healthy desserts, snacks, shakes, and other foods, sweetened with honey or fruit to maintain a low glycemic index.

Although buying raw, organic cocoa for your recipes is the obvious choice, avoiding highly processed types is also important. This includes cocoa labeled "processed with alkali," which is also known as Dutch processing or Dutching. It might sound sexy, but this kind of cocoa contains significantly reduced levels of phytonutrients—up to 90 percent less flavonoids.

Real, unsweetened cocoa typically contains significant protein content of about 7 or 8 grams per ounce. It is also low in carbohydrate—between 8 and 13 grams per ounce, with 50 to 60 percent or more of that carbohydrate coming in the form of fiber. Like other beans, cocoa contains many vitamins and minerals, including natural folates, niacin, zinc, and magnesium.

About half of the content of cocoa is natural fat. This cocoa butter also has great health benefits, with great taste a key reason it's so delicious. While it can be used to make white chocolate, there is little to no flavonoids in cocoa fat.

Cocoa butter does have nutritional attributes. More than a third of it is health-promoting monounsaturated oil, and it contains the essential fatty acid linoleic acid. It also has a moderate amount of stearic acid. Though saturated, this fat can help reduce LDL cholesterol. Because of its strong antioxidant ingredients, cocoa can protect us against LDL-cholesterol damage.

Is cocoa addicting? Many people are aware of the intense craving they have for chocolate. But the high levels of added sugar contained in most products are probably more addictive than the cocoa alone. However, psychoactive compounds present in cocoa, salsolinol being the main one, might be why chocolate itself can be addicting. Also, a typical single serving of cocoa may contain 25 to 50 mg of caffeine (compared to a cup of coffee, which can have 100 to 300 mg, and black tea's 50 to 140 mg of caffeine), enough for many people to notice a buzz.

The flavonoids and polyphenols in cocoa are much like those in grape skins. This might make cocoa the next red wine as research trends continue unlocking its many health mysteries.

Update on Dairy

Another common question I receive from athletes is about dairy foods. Are they part of a healthy diet? While I've addressed many aspects of this topic in past articles and books, there is both a short and long answer—the focus of this update.

The short answers about dairy are that it depends on the individual and whether they can tolerate these products, and on the ability to find healthy versions of these foods. While dairy can be a healthy part of a great diet for some people, for many others, it can wreck the body's immune system, gut, and even the brain.

The long answer is more complex. The most important factor is that there are two general types of dairy products: those that can be healthy for certain people, and others that should be avoided by everyone. This idea rules out most of the dairy products available to consumers, narrowing down the healthy possibilities. To further sort out the dairy dos and don'ts, below are specific issues to consider, which include low-quality dairy (junk food), individuality, lactose and fermented foods, and milk proteins.

Low Quality Dairy—Junk Food

Most dairy products come from the milk of unhealthy cows, goats, or sheep. These source animals are not cared for in a humane and healthy way, and are usually treated with antibiotics, hormones, and exposed to other chemicals that can find their way into the milk and products made from it. Despite the use of antibiotics, much of this milk does not pass inspection as grade "A." However, this milk is still sold to consumers, as grade "C" dried milk. It's used in many packaged food products, including powdered milk. All these dairy products get my grade of "junk food" and should always be avoided. Go into any grocery store and whether it's a container of milk, cheese, or many packaged products containing dried milk, it's an unhealthy choice. Many are also found in health food stores. This rules out the majority of all dairy products.

The healthiest dairy foods would include products made from certified organic animals that are grass fed and well cared for. While these may be available in stores, they are more easily found in local farms or farmer's markets, where the person who milked the cow or at least someone familiar with the farm is often there to ask about quality.

Individuality

I'm shocked that some people continually consume foods that don't agree with them. It's sometimes a minor symptom of indigestion or a slight brain fog following ingestion. While these feelings are often very minor, other people feel downright ill after eating dairy foods—headaches, nausea, skin rashes, and others—clear indications that the food should strictly be avoided. Obviously, these individuals should avoid all dairy products.

Others don't seem to have any signs or symptoms after consuming dairy. However, this does not always mean the food is good for you.

The easiest way to determine if dairy is causing any problems is to strictly avoid it for a period of ten days to two weeks. Before you start, write down any problems you might have, whether you think they're related to dairy or not, from minor physical aches or fatigue, to sleeping problems and skin- or hair-related signs. After your period without dairy, re-evaluate your list to see if anything has changed. If there's a noticeable difference, most likely the dairy was a stress on your body. Otherwise, add the same amount of dairy you were previously eating and see if there's a worsening of any signs or symptoms, or the creation of new problems. If this is the case, dairy may not be for you.

Sometimes, dairy can be part of a complex pattern of problems in the body and often cause secondary signs or symptoms. For example, people who are allergic or sensitive to wheat or refined carbohydrates often have dairy-related symptoms, too. But let's say wheat is a primary problem and dairy secondary, avoiding all wheat may eliminate the secondary sensitivity to dairy.

Another individuality issue has to do with overall health. Those who are healthiest can more often digest and absorb nutrients from dairy much better and without distress than those who are unhealthy.

Just what parts of dairy cause trouble for those sensitive or allergic? It depends on the person, but lactose (milk sugar) and casein (milk protein) are two common culprits.

Lactose and Fermented Foods

A major component of milk is the sugar lactose, which poses a potential problem for many consumers. While a good number of people have difficulty digesting lactose, others cannot digest it at all. In order to digest lactose, an enzyme called lactase is required, which digests the complex lactose into simple sugars. Without adequate digestion, lactose can ferment in the intestine, producing gas, bloating, cramps, and diarrhea. Lactose-digestion problems are also associated with more serious disorders such as irritable bowel syndrome, and symptoms beyond the gut such as premenstrual syndrome, headaches, fatigue, mental depression, and others.

Because of its relatively high lactose content, drinking milk, especially for adults and many children, is best avoided.

Many people who have problems with cow milk find that they can sometimes tolerate milk from sheep and goats much better because these may be lower in lactose. The fat in both goat and sheep milk is made up of smaller fat globules that also are easier to digest.

The problem of lactose can be remedied by using the process of fermentation, where healthy bacteria are added to milk to make cheese, yogurt, and kefir. This can significantly reduce the amount of lactose in these products because the bacteria consume lactose for food.

For many people, these fermented dairy products can be healthy, especially when made from the milk of organic, grass-fed animals. A variety of cheeses, yogurt, and kefir are dairy products that come without many of the lactose-related problems associated with liquid milk. These cheeses can be found in many stores, local farms and markets, and on the Internet, and they're easy to make at home.

Consumer, beware:

- Avoid the fruit-flavored and sweetened varieties of yogurt and kefir that are usually full of sugar—sometimes with a half-dozen teaspoons or more. Buy the plain variety and if necessary, add fresh fruit or small amounts of honey.
- In addition, avoid so-called "American" cheese, cheese spreads, and other processed cheeses. These highly refined products, which outsell natural cheese, are usually made from several types of unripe cheeses, ground up with added chemical stabilizers, preservatives, and emulsifiers. Some are even organic, an example of the rapidly growing "organic junk food" segment of the so-called health food industry.

It's important to remember that dairy is also high in saturated fat. But the makeup of this fat depends on the diet of the animal. This is another reason to only consume dairy from grass fed animals, which has a better quality of saturated fatty acids.

Unlike earlier studies, recent research indicates that dairy fat may not significantly contribute to chronic inflammation. However, it's still important to consider the balance of dietary fats to assure one avoids the overproduction of inflammatory chemicals. (For the average person, avoiding vegetable oils and consuming adequate cold-water fish or fish oil capsules is more important than the amount of dairy fat consumed.)

The best cheese is produced with raw milk, like the traditional cheeses made for centuries (the same way it's done in Europe today).

Milk Proteins

Remember Little Miss Muffet, eating her curds and whey? These are the two proteins found in milk. Whey protein is the thin liquid part of milk remaining after the curds—called casein—are removed.

Whey is the part of the milk containing most of the vitamins and minerals, including calcium, and it's a complete protein. During the making of cheese, which mostly is produced from curds, whey is often fed back to the animals for nutritional reasons. However, making whey cheese, called ricotta, from fresh raw milk is a great option. When buying it, check the label and make sure whey, not curds, is the main ingredient (many cheap ricotta products are made with whole milk and not whey).

Whey is also made into powders for use in baked goods, energy bars, and smoothies. If you're using powdered whey, buy organic.

The whey component of milk is also healthy because it contains a group of natural sulfur-containing substances called biothiols that help produce the main antioxidant in our cells called gluta-thione. Because it helps the immune system, whey has been used in the treatment of many chronic conditions, from asthma and allergies to cancer and heart disease. It can also help improve muscle function.

Most people who are allergic to cow's milk can usually consume whey without problems. Small amounts of lactose are found in whey (much less than is found in liquid milk) but this is usually too little to cause intestinal problems, even in most people who are a bit sensitive to lactose. In those who are truly lactose-intolerant (probably less than 5 percent of the population), this amount of lactose could be a problem.

The curds from milk are used for most cheese making. Cottage cheese is the best example of what curds look like. However, it's the curd that most people are allergic to when there's a dairy allergy. Newborns and young children are particularly vulnerable to curds because their intestine and immune system are too immature to tolerate this protein.

But not all casein is the same. Two of the most common types are called "A1" and "A2." As a protein, A1 behaves like an opiate and has been associated with chronic illness and disease; but A2 has not. If you consume dairy products, it's important to further narrow your choices to those made from milk with little or no A1.

Research shows a strong association between the consumption of A1 casein and various health problems. Numerous studies, including data from the World Health Organization (WHO), have linked A1 with increased risk of heart disease, high cholesterol, diabetes, sudden infant death syndrome, and neurological disorders, such as autism and schizophrenia. These health issues are not associated with consumption of A2 casein.

Most people think of black and white cows as the source of their milk. These animals, called Holsteins (the U.S. breed) and Friesians (the European version), are the most common sources of milk on the market. These large, high volume milk producers are most commonly used by big corporate dairy farms. They are typically given bST (bovine somatotropin—a hormone used to increases the cow's milk production), and provided with special feeds of corn and synthetic vitamins rather than grass. These animals produce milk that contains higher amounts of beta-casein type A1. (Reddish colored cows, including Ayrshire and Milking Short Horns, are also in this category and less common.)

The other types of dairy cows are smaller, and brownish and white in color. These are called Jersey, Guernsey, and Brown Swiss cows. They produce lesser volumes of milk, are naturally resistant to disease, and convert grass to milk quite efficiently. These animals produce milk containing predominantly A2 casein—the healthy type. Their milk is similar to that of other animals including goat, sheep, buffalo, yaks, donkeys, and camels—milk from these animals contain mostly A2 and little A1.

How can you tell which type of animal your milk comes from? Unfortunately, in most cases, the milk from many different herds of cows are mixed by the time it gets to the store as milk or cheese. This makes it impossible to tell what you're getting regarding the kinds of casein it contains. The best way to purchase this milk, or the products made from it, is at the farm, co-op, or farmer's market, where you can often buy raw milk or cheese, and find out what types of cows are producing it.

If all this sounds complicated, it may be. Finding healthy dairy products is getting more difficult. However, by looking locally, even in large cities where country farmers are coming in for weekend markets, it's getting easier to find these foods.

Like with many food items in today's marketplace, the majority of dairy products should be avoided. I consume dairy regularly. This includes a variety of cheeses, sour cream, and butter, all made with fresh raw milk from organic, well-fed, and humanely treated animals.

The Search for Healthy Food

Many people who are new to buying and preparing fresh healthy foods face a huge challenge: where to find it? Those of us who have sought healthy food for years and decades know the routine of hunting through stores, farmer's markets, and our own backyards. I am fortunately to have homegrown fresh food all year long, including chickens for eggs, cheese from raw milk, and find local meats that are beyond organic.

Look for Local Family Farms

Fortunately for most people, there's an abundance of healthy food nearby, but it may take some searching initially. Consider a small family farm—here are some I've eaten from:

- In Colorado, the local *Arkansas* Valley *Organic* Growers is one example, with great vegetables and meats.
- The Ohio Ecological Food and Farm Association was a great find.
- Small family farms in the Catskill Mountains are gaining in popularity, providing great vegetables, eggs, and meats.

With these and other local farms, millions of people can find healthy food more easily than ever.

Check out Localharvest.org for a listing of various types of local food. Beware: just because they claim to be homegrown, make sure they are, and that they're organic or otherwise all natural. Visiting the farm to see for yourself is worth a trip.

With the problems in the organic industry, including the easing of a strict standard in growing and producing the cleanest and highest quality foods, and the added bureaucratic costs due to the certification process, many truly health-conscious consumers are looking at this choice. Farmers markets are now part of the urban landscape, attracting weekend crowds. There are community organic cooperatives, roadside farm stands, and "pick-your-own" fruit and vegetable farms. These modern markets feature products grown in a "green" way—produced in line with the original organic movement. And, they often include a "buy local" slogan.

But the underlying problem is that there is no regulation regarding whether it's "green," organic, or beyond organic. One problem is the notion that products that are better than organic— the "beyond organic" movement—should be more expensive. But just because products are grown with care, without chemicals, doesn't mean they should be more expensive. Without the "middlemen"—typically two, three, or more of them taking a share before products get to the retail stores—most of these products should be less expensive than the same or similar products in retail stores.

If you're a careful consumer and talk to the farmers and those producing these products, and even visit their farms, you can usually find high-quality healthy products that are often better than the organic version in retail stores, often for less cost. Supply and demand will help "weed out" the overpriced products.

Growing Your Own

One option most people have is to grow some, or even most, of their own food. Surprisingly, it can be done easily, inexpensively, and legally, even in a very small piece of backyard or indoors. "Right to farm" laws in all states are now in effect, so don't let anyone tell you that chickens or planting is illegal.

Most "right to farm" laws were enacted in the 1980s and today all U.S. states have them. It gives individuals the right to grow food, raise chickens, and other animals, and to pursue other related activities. These laws do not give farmers complete freedom to do as they please, but they offer protection from local ordinances claiming "chickens are not allowed" and other restrictions. Farmers must operate in a legal and reasonable manner to be eligible for the law's protection.

In many states, right-to-farm laws supersede even local laws that might run contrary to them. In Pennsylvania, for instance, state law mandates that every municipality in the state "encourage the continuity, development and viability of agricultural operations within its jurisdiction," regardless of whatever local laws may arise in opposition to this mandate.

Lawn to Garden

Tens of millions of people farm the wrong kind of crop: grass. It often costs a lot but does not return anything other than having a nice green turf around the home. Putting that money into planting a garden would return many times that dollar amount in healthy, delicious food.

Ted Steinberg, author of *"American Green: The Obsessive Quest for the Perfect Lawn," says that the lawn is one of America's leading crops with up to forty million acres of turf.*

Unfortunately, because of the way they're maintained, many lawns are also toxic to the environment. "Lawns use ten times as many chemicals per acre as industrial farmland. These pesticides, fertilizers, and herbicides run off into our groundwater and evaporate into our air, causing widespread pollution and global warming, and greatly increasing our risk of cancer, heart disease, and birth defects," writes Heather Coburn Flores, author of the book *Food Not Lawns*. She says that the pollution emitted from a power mower in just one hour is equal to the amount from a car being driven 350 miles. And, Flores says, U.S. lawns consume around 270 billion gallons of water a week, which may be enough to grow eighty million acres of organic vegetables. Using part (or all) of your lawn to grow food is easier than you think. To research this idea, Google these topics:

- Square foot gardening
- Lasagna gardening
- SPIN (small plot intensive) gardening
- Bio-intensive gardening
- No till/no dig gardening

Food is what powers our body to be the best endurance athletes. Don't cheat your body and brain by eating junk food. Get into the habit of only buying healthy food—then it's less likely to find its way into your house.

CHILDREN ARE CHAMPIONS

Development of the human athlete starts before birth as I described in Section 5. Newborns quickly continue building both health and fitness, and should be given every opportunity to move, without physical restriction. Training continues through infancy, during which children naturally want to be involved with a variety of activities.

Unfortunately, the process of development more often does not go as nature intends. Our modern society actually *discourages* children from growing into great endurance athletes. This is done through increased screen time—TV and computer games, to name two distractions—restriction of movements, especially during early years, along with the consumption of junk food, too often baby's first formula meal.

Instead, emphasis should be on making room for the roaming infant's journey in the best environment, letting them crawl, walk and run, climb and jump to their desires (as long as it's safe, of course). A wide variety of physical movements are vital parts of neuromuscular progress, and necessities for the brain, with early physical activity ultimately making the child better at math, science, music, coordination, and social skills.

While great health and fitness during childhood may lead to great athletic performance later in life, a key reason children's fitness is important is this: *Fitness is widely recognized as a powerful marker of current and future cardiovascular, musculoskeletal, and mental health.*

The process of childhood training, of course, is different than that of adult athletes. Children's activities need a wide range of movement for their innate talents will evolve. As they grow through the first decade of life, natural development will lead to various interests regarding specific activities. But they still are not ready for adult endurance training, which involves specialization, steady state, and schedules.

Easier said than done as parents, uncles, neighbors, and others who may have some degree of sports knowledge may want to intervene and help push the process along. While some children normally develop at faster rates and others at a slower pace, we can't really predict who will ultimately be great in a group of young school-aged athletes, whether ten, thirteen, sixteen, or any age. Pushing children into training may seem helpful, but if the young athlete is not on board, the process will be impaired—another negative lifestyle that could even lead to the common casualty of an inactive, overweight child.

There are two important keys when it comes to children transitioning to adolescent athletes:

- *Cross training.* From before birth through age twenty or so, the whole body undergoes dramatic changes. Of utmost importance is the physical activity that plays a key role in this process—the more variety of movement, the better the development. This contributes to muscle and bone growth, hormone balance, immune function, and brain maturation. At certain ages, selected sports activities may draw certain interests—riding a bike, swimming, running, soccer, and other games—but variety continues to be important.

- The second feature is simple—the process of having active fun. It may be the most important guideline for children.

Unfortunately, generations of children have quickly learned that watching TV, playing video games, and being *inactive* is the new form of fun. Studies confirm it, showing that their fitness has been failing for decades, as they continue getting fatter.

Children's Fitness is Declining

In the United States, the endurance performance of children continues to decline. The American Heart Association reports that this reduction occurred at a rate of about 6 percent per decade between 1970 and 2000. The rest of the world is following in pursuit, with all children about 15 percent less fit than their parents were when they were young.

Overall, in a one-mile run, today's children are about a minute and a half slower than their peers thirty years ago.

Many children can't run as far or fast as their parents did, according to research presented at the American Heart Association's (AHA) Scientific Sessions in November 2013. "If a young person is generally unfit now, then they are more likely to develop conditions like heart disease later in life," said Grant Tomkinson, PhD, lead author of the study and senior lecturer in the University of South Australia's School of Health Sciences.

The decline in endurance may predict diminished health in adulthood, the researchers said.

Researchers analyzed fifty studies on running fitness between 1964 and 2010 that involved more than twenty-five million children ages nine to seventeen from twenty-eight countries. They defined endurance by how far kids could run in a set time or distance with tests typically lasting five to fifteen minutes or a half-mile to two miles. Researchers showed that endurance declined significantly within the forty-six years, with average changes similar between boys and girls, younger and older kids, and across different regions.

The study is the first to show that kids' cardiovascular fitness has declined around the globe since about 1975. Here are more sad statistics:

- In the U.S., children's endurance fell an average 6 percent per decade between 1970 and 2000.
- Throughout the world, endurance declined consistently by about 5 percent per decade.
- Today's children are roughly 15 percent less fit than their parents were as youngsters.

The AHA confirmed an obvious relationship, showing the connection between poor fitness and being overfat, with childhood obesity rates tripling since the 1980. Tomkinson said the children should engage in at least sixty minutes of daily activities that use the body's big muscles, such as running, swimming, or cycling, and that, "We need to help to inspire children and youth to develop fitness habits that will keep them healthy now and into the future."

Among the side effects of poor fitness is that, for the first time in history, the youngest generation is set to have a shorter lifespan than their parents.

Diminishing endurance in children, and their high level of overfatness, including babies, is obviously a major problem. And it is no doubt connected with adults—in the U.S. up to 75 percent of them are overfat. This epidemic continues to grow in all people despite the $60 billion annual weight-loss industry, the White House Task Force on Childhood Obesity, and many other approaches, all of which have failed to a great degree because the *causes* of the problem are not addressed. Among them are junk food as the daily diet, and an emphasis of inactivity even in schools.

Organized Sports

As young children get into puberty, where hormones play a huge role in developing their physical and mental bodies, various team and individual sports opportunities arise.

In time, many children will want to get involved with organized sports, whether it be independent activities such as swimming, biking, or running, a team sport such as little league baseball, or casual activities with friends walking, biking, or skate boarding. Young children want to have fun, and this is the approach that should be maintained—even through adulthood.

Injuries

More than thirty million children participate in sports. Unfortunately, injuries are common whether it's from biking, running, racquet sports, baseball, or basketball. Over a third of all school-aged children sustain injuries severe enough to warrant a visit to a health-care practitioner, with many more injured who don't seek professional assistance. Many children can create silent problems that may not produce symptoms for months or even years. A seemingly minor muscle imbalance, for example, can easily become chronic. This can significantly affect growth, and then posture and gait, and may even contribute to injuries in adulthood. Of course, shoes are the biggest culprit here, an important issue discussed in Section 4.

Because a variety of physical activities are so important in childhood (and even for adults), multisport activities are ideal. Being involved in different kinds of activities, and those that change with the seasons, will keep a child's brain and body most balanced

As children become ready for friendly competition, events such as the triathlon are ideal due to its variety of swimming, biking, and running. However, long events of any type are best avoided until children are older.

The main risk for children performing three (or more) events is overdoing it. But like adults, a large volume of training is not necessarily best. Keep it simple, and keep it short. Most importantly, keep it fun.

In addition, virtually all the concerns about adults who train also apply to children. These include avoiding overtraining, including injuries, diet and nutrition, sports shoes, heart rate monitors, and other factors such as the need for an active warm-up and cool down. A study in the *Journal of Exercise Physiology* (2006), for example, showed that an active warm-up can significantly influence performance in children, and that static stretching may be detrimental in preparing children for activities.

An important aspect of sports for children is letting them learn on their own, sometimes with your help. Young athletes who are physically active from a very early age are often seen reading books on sports. This offers an ideal scenario for learning, teaching, developing, and having fun.

My Perspective by Coralee Thompson, MD

As a mother and physician, I never pushed organized sports on my two sons, although we exercised together almost every day. By six years old and every fall until age thirteen, they would participate in their grade school-sponsored triathlon that included a four hundred-meter swim, ten kilometers of biking, and five kilometers of running.

Throughout the year, we would swim two or three times a week and run at least four days a week. These workouts were always slow and easy. While running, the boys would wear heart rate monitors to make sure their heart rates did not exceed 165 beats per minute. We had fun being together and feeling the positive effects of exercise. As soon as school finished, we would start biking together on park trails. The focus was having fun, while gradually increasing the distance of successive rides.

Two month before the race we would start putting two different exercises together, for example—run and then swim. The most difficult transition was always biking followed by running. No matter how easy we would bike, our legs felt like jelly in the beginning of the run. By one month before the triathlon, every day included two exercises together. Two weeks before the event, we did a mock trial.

The triathlon was a joyful experience among their classmates, teachers, and parents. When finishing the event, each kid would continue running with younger classmates still racing until everyone had finished. As a parent, my greatest satisfaction was not the results of the triathlons—but rather our consistent exercise time together.

Children and Healthy Food

It's never too early to encourage a healthy diet. As adults with healthy habits, we can influence children in a positive way from the time they are born. The other way is that we allow others to have negative unhealthy influences. These problems come in the form of unhealthy traditions, such as feeding babies processed cereal, giving unhealthy desserts as reward, allowing candy from relatives and friends, and even allowing treats at the dentist or doctor's office.

Basically, all the recommendations I've made in this and other books can apply to children after weaning. (For more information see the book *Healthy Brains Healthy Children*, or visit the Healthy Children pages at www.philmaffetone.com.)

The sad news is that most of today's children will be part of tomorrow's overfat epidemic sufferers. A young child who learns to be physically active achieves only part of the protection that can prevent this problem. The other is eating well. As parents know, just working out does not make one immune to the building of fat stores—it takes both proper physical activity and a healthy diet.

When it comes to children's eating habits we all know they are easily influenced from friends, their parents, and other adults. Most frightening is how vulnerable young people are to advertisements and media hype—much of which comes from TV. So it's more important to counter that propaganda with proper habits and healthy, rational discussions, beginning at a very early age. Helping in the kitchen, planting a garden, and shopping for healthy food at any age helps children understand the importance of natural foods.

Children who are most vulnerable to blood sugar problems generally have a certain history. The items below apply to those most susceptible to carbohydrate intolerance:

- Low or high birth weight (5½ pounds or less, nine points or more)
- Taller than average for age
- Increased weight or body fat
- Sleep problems
- Mother: increased stress during pregnancy
- Increased aggression or anger
- Attention-deficit hyperactive disorder (ADHD)
- Physical activity low
- Family history: diabetes, high blood pressure, high cholesterol or triglycerides, heart disease or stroke, breast cancer

These signs and symptoms do not necessarily mean your child is destined to have blood sugar irregularities. Making appropriate changes discussed throughout this book can significantly reduce and often eliminate these problems.

Young Athlete's Feet

There's really not much to say about children's feet. Almost all are perfect at birth, and they continue to be a marvel of anatomy until a shoe is placed on it. The more children remain naturally barefoot, the healthier their feet will develop. And, the less they rely on footwear, the longer into adulthood their feet will remain healthy.

For most sports, some type of shoe is needed. Keep them flat, simple, and comfortable. The same aspects as those for adult shoes (discussed in Section 4) apply to children's shoes. Unfortunately, foot and shoe related injuries occur in children much the same way as in adults. The ankle and knee are the most common areas in which injuries occur in children. Most of the knee injuries are non-traumatic, meaning they are secondary to some other problem—mostly caused by shoes. In addition, most with non-trauma knee pain may have foot problems, often those that are asymptomatic, that caused the knee problem.

First Feet

Brimming with powerful nerve endings, a baby's feet are an opportunity to stimulate healthy neurological and physical development from the earliest age. Easy massage or even just simple regular rubbing of the feet can be potent therapeutic actions. Children of any age can benefit from this to prevent future problems.

Preventive strategies are best implemented early in life. In this case, taking advantage of the easily accessible and effective ways to improve health through stimulation of the bottoms of the baby's feet is helpful.

Children most often have normal feet but they don't always look like adult feet. As children start walking, they may even appear flat-footed. This is due to the baby fat that is not only in their face and belly, but also in the arches of their feet. This physiologic flatfoot appearance should not be confused with a pathologic flatfoot condition. Myths about this phenomenon are sometimes perpetuated by health professionals, shoe companies, popular magazines, and even the media.

A pathologic flatfoot condition is one in which the foot and ankle are very rigid, but this is rare. Many children have normal physiologically flat feet, and eventually the feet form a normal, healthy arch. Unfortunately, too many children with physiologic flatfeet are treated for abnormal conditions, often with supports, bracing, or special shoes. This can be ineffective and, as studies show, can put significant psychological stress on the child, especially those in school. If your health care professional recommends some type of therapy for your child's feet, consider getting one or more additional opinions, including optional therapies.

My Perspective by Judy Hetkowski

As a middle school physical education teacher, trying to instill the importance of healthy exercise and other aspects of fitness was a challenge. But having been a patient of Dr. Phil's, learning by example helped make the process of working with children more successful and enjoyable.

I started my middle school physical education students running slow at the first part of class as a warm-up and for aerobic conditioning. Everyone ran the six hundred-meter loop around the outdoor field, and many of the students went more than the required one lap—because they wanted to. We encouraged the students to go slowly to stay aerobic. This approach was a challenge for young boys and girls. By this point in their lives, the faster-is-better mentally was already in place. Going slower to go longer was a difficult concept, but the enjoyment quickly was realized for most of them. Soon, our students were running farther than the high school girls who were training for long distance events.

Our cross country/track program for seventh and eighth grade girls had well over fifty runners. In addition to being the largest team around, we had an additional benefit: we continued to emphasize good health and fitness, including warming up, training slow, and cooling down. We developed many talented runners.

Until I became a patient of Dr. Phil's, my own previous running history had been a constant struggle. I was always hurt and could never run more than fifteen miles a week without injury.

At first I thought Phil was a witch doctor, but before I knew it my chronic injuries were gone and he helped me become physically and mentally healthy. In addition, he coached me so I could train without injury or illness. I remember one of the first things he told me: You're trying to be fit before you're healthy. It was at this point that I started to compete, and also refine my teaching and coaching at school.

The heart rate training and dietary advice greatly helped me. It also allowed me to apply the same information to coaching and teaching my students, which was emphasizing individuality— every student was uniquely different.

When our first group of junior-high girls graduated to high school, there was no team for them, and we had to find funding for a high-school team. In its first year we were the Section One champions, and went on to finish third overall in New York State. Many of the girls continued on with their health-and-fitness habits after high school.

In health classes, I began addressing many issues about food. For example, we brought in food packages and learned about ingredients, teaching that the less the number of ingredients the better and not to eat things with ingredients they couldn't pronounce. The students kept a diary of the foods and the portions they had for an evaluation of their own diets. I also encouraged students not on the running teams to participate in the after-school 50/100-mile endurance club.

My own training continued to improve. I was able to run farther and faster at the same heart rates. While some fellow runners chuckled at my very slow warm-ups, slow training, and wearing a heart monitor, I suddenly began racing faster than many of them. Over a period of time, my racing improved dramatically, and when I reached the master's level I was suddenly a top-ranked American master's runner.

One of the few master's women runners who always outper-formed me was my new friend, and also a patient of Dr. Phil's, England's Priscilla Welch (and who was the first woman in the 1987 New York City marathon at age forty-two).

I was fortunate to earn many gold medals at the National Master's events from 5K to 15K on the roads and in cross-country throughout the country. I also won a bronze medal overall in the World Veterans 10K Championship.

Phil's lessons were invaluable to me personally and to my teaching and coaching, and remain so today. Almost 30 years later, I continue to run daily, and practice the same good workout and nutrition.

Pregnant Athletes

While I've discussed the before-birth experience of the youngest athletes, the mothers are athletic too. How can pregnant women train? The short answer, of course, is by being healthy and fit. Comfort during any particular activity should also be a priority. Swimming is always a great option, but only in clean, open water or a salt pool. (Pregnant women should avoid chlorine.) There have also been plenty of women who compete as well, and some who have run marathons and longer distances while pregnant.

30-plus Years of Pregnant Marathons by Tracy Høeg MD, PhD

The first marathon run by a pregnant woman might have been in 1983. And, not surprisingly, it was unintentional. The Norwegian Ingrid Christiansen ran the Houston Marathon in 2:33:27 and was disappointed with her time. It wasn't until two months later her coach, Johan Kaggestad, suggested she perform a pregnancy test. She was 5 feet, 6 inches, 106 pounds and used to infrequent periods. She called her coach crying. The test was positive. It wasn't that she didn't want to get pregnant; she did. But she also wanted to continue running. She ran around 200km per week the first two months of pregnancy.

Just to give a little historical perspective, in 1966, Roberta Gibb had her entry form for the Boston Marathon returned with a note that stated women were "not physically capable" of running a marathon. She ran anyway, thus disproving the theory of the author of the note.

Certainly there were women capable of running a marathon, though they were the exceptional few who had trained enough to be capable. As early as the 1930s, scientists and physicians discussed the safety of exercise during pregnancy. Smaller studies were done on animals and women, but by today's rigorous research standards, nothing significant was deduced. In the 1980s, evidence escalated that some degree of exercise and/or running was acceptable and was likely to be beneficial. This was reflected in the American College of Obstetricians and Gynecologists' 1985 exercise in pregnancy guidelines. And today healthy women are usually advised they can continue training at the same level they trained at prior to pregnancy.

In 2012 more than 200,000 women completed marathons in the United States alone. This does not take into account the number of women who completed long-distance triathlons or ultramarathons. Many of these women are in their child-bearing years and will be interested to know if they can continue this type of racing and training while pregnant.

A careful reader might deduce: if a woman is currently allowed to continue training at her current level when she becomes pregnant and she is in the shape to run a marathon prior to pregnancy, then she can run one pregnant.

Is it indeed this simple?

Once the words pregnancy and marathon are combined, the general public disapproves. Of course, they view the marathon through the eyes of a person who is not in the condition to run a marathon, perhaps let alone a 5k, so it simply *seems* too dangerous. And women who are pregnant read the thoughts of these people and get discouraged.

But in March of 2013, the *American Journal of Family Practice* became part of an official movement of not discouraging women from running marathons pregnant. The article states recreational athletes can continue to train at their current level in an uncomplicated pregnancy.

The concerns about running a marathon pregnant are speculative and few.

- Is there an increased risk of miscarriage?
- Would the core body temperature of a marathoner rise to such a degree that it poses a risk to the fetus's central nervous system? And if so, at what point in pregnancy?
- Does the transient decreased heart rate observed in fetuses while a mother is running pose a risk? Or does it in fact make the baby's cardiovascular system stronger and more resilient?

Studies with small populations and large epidemiological studies with multiple confounding variables have not been able to either confirm or debunk these concerns.

In the meantime, many women are running marathons pregnant. So why is it you may have only heard of Amber Miller and perhaps one or two others? Because actually, it's not really big news for runners. At nearly every large city marathon, there are one or more women running it pregnant. They may choose to announce it on a blog, Facebook, or simply tell friends. But the press rarely gets word.

I love looking at pregnant runners. Is there another point in a woman's life when she simply glows? Some of the best running experiences I have had were when I was pregnant. The distance and speed you run at is up to you. Remember, there are so many health benefits for both you and your baby. Your own happiness is among the most important.

When I became pregnant in 2007, I just kept running—some 13 miles a day. I wrote about it on my blog, and only because readers started voicing concerns did I start researching it. I soon learned that most of what you find online is from women (and men) discouraging women from continuing to run because it is too *selfish* (this is a word that will break any pregnant woman's heart). Even *The Girlfriend's Guide to Pregnancy* by Vicki Iovine discourages women from engaging in any exercise whatsoever while pregnant.

These non-scientifically sound opinions are doing a true disservice to women athletes (and really all women), who are interested in having a healthy, happy pregnancy.

Subsequent to my pregnancy, I found a woman online who had run seven marathons pregnant. Her website has now disappeared and I don't remember her name—perhaps she had threats from her readers of contacting the police, as I did on my blog. Then I heard about a woman who had reportedly run a Midwest ultramarathon while nine months pregnant. I heard it from two different people who don't know each other. Yet, I wonder if the legend created around her is larger than her belly got. This is just the nature of pregnant marathon "evidence." Women don't want to *brag* about running pregnant. They just want to do it and not cause any trouble.

By 2010, I had heard of or read about nearly fifty women who had run marathons pregnant. I never heard of complications. And I had read *Exercising Through Your Pregnancy* by James F. Clapp III, MD, which demonstrated through elegant research not only how safe running while pregnant was, but also the myriad benefits to the mother and baby that go along with running during the entire pregnancy. These include much lower rates of pregnancy complications and health benefits for the child including better self-calming, decreased chance of obesity, improved motor coordination, and higher IQ. So one is led to wonder: would running a lot result in an ideal pregnancy and a super child? Or is there a point where it gets risky?

That same year, I was contacted by a "Ms. S" who had read my running blog. She had a few questions and wanted to know about my experience running while pregnant. She went on to set a personal record (PR) in the half-marathon while four months pregnant, and then another PR in the marathon while six months pregnant—finishing in 3:27. I was floored. Not only did running a marathon pregnant now appear to be safe, but also running one at a higher speed than achieved pre-pregnancy was safe for at least this woman. It should be pointed out, though, that she suffered a stress fracture late in pregnancy, and these are the types of issues that need to be further explored so women can avoid injury to their rapidly changing bodies.

In the summer of 2010, I became pregnant again. I continued training at an intense level. I had a fifty-mile race on my schedule when I was six weeks pregnant. I ran the race at a comfortable pace and felt surprisingly good the entire time. I had, though, run the race the year before an hour faster. The very next day, before I went to bed, I noticed pink in my underwear. By the next morning, I was bleeding so heavily that I knew it was a miscarriage. I blamed myself and the fifty-mile race entirely. But I made the very wise decision to go to the hospital. They did an ultrasound there, which ended up making a lot more sense: the fetus had died three weeks earlier. Whether or not it had anything to do with a high level of training, I probably will never know.

But that fall, I got pregnant again. I ran six marathons during that pregnancy and gave birth to a healthy boy at thirty-nine weeks. I ran the first marathon just three weeks pregnant (before the pregnancy test turned positive) and I was noticeably winded compared to my most recent marathon. My last pregnant marathon was the Copenhagen Marathon at thirty weeks pregnant, which I ran in 4:54. After that very strenuous effort, I had a long recovery and lots of Braxton Hicks contractions. I had to wonder how healthy such a fast marathon at thirty weeks was in retrospect. But in the end, I have no doubt that running while pregnant was the right thing for me, as it is for many other women.

And what about Ingrid Christiansen? What happened to her after all of those kilometers and a world-class marathon time two months pregnant? She had an uncomplicated pregnancy and gave birth to a healthy baby boy. Just six months later, she went on to set the women's marathon world record in 2:24:26 in London in 1984. She lowered it again by three minutes a year later.

Improved performance post-partum is a less discussed "benefit" of running while pregnant, but worth mentioning for moms-to-be who want to continue running. In the small amount of literature written about the *doping* effect of pregnancy, young women athletes in Eastern Germany during the 1970s are mentioned and it was termed "abortion doping." Supposedly these women got pregnant simply to induce red blood cell production and then would abort the baby and get a boost in their training similar to what one would get with EPO (Erythropoietin) doping—imagine training in such a malignant environment! (This effect should not last more than three months, given the life of a red blood cell.)

But time and again, I have witnessed and heard of women who have gone on to set personal records in running all sorts of distances after (an entire) pregnancy, though not within the first three months post-partum. So there must be a more long-lasting form of "doping" and I think the answer may lie in muscle memory.

The body simply adjusts to all of that extra weight and when that weight is suddenly gone, the mother's body is much more efficient at running. I do not know how long this lasts, but suspect it is between one and two years and is likely more pronounced the more you run while pregnant. And of course, if you continue to train, you can extend the benefits out for many years.

In the past, health care providers instructed women to wait six weeks after delivery to begin exercising. But in an uncomplicated, vaginal delivery, women may now begin running again within days of delivery—entirely up to their own level of comfort—if they can find the time!

Tracy Høeg started long-distance running when she was seventeen, after no longer having a basketball or soccer team to run with. She used running to help her stay healthy and battle stress during college and medical school. It was her future husband who convinced her to start racing when she was twenty-seven. Tracy upped her running mileage significantly during her first pregnancy and was surprised by both the positive and negative reactions she received while running and racing pregnant. She has written extensively about women's issues in running at her personal blog http:// sealegsgirl.blogspot.com/ and is a long-distance running health writer at irunfar.com. She is a post-doc fellow at the University of Copenhagen and currently researches vision loss, ultramarathon-induced vision loss, training at maximum aerobic function training (MAF), and has for a number of years collected data on women who continue to run competitively during pregnancy. She was also a member of Team USA at the World Championships in Ultra Trail Running in 2013. In 2015, she will begin medical specialty training in Physical Medicine and Rehabilitation at the University of California-Irvine.

Children are our next generation of champions—not only in sports but in making the world a healthier and a more fit place to be.

AGE, ATHLETICS, AND GROWING YOUNGER

The ageless Hall of Fame baseball pitcher Satchel Paige said it best: "How old would you be if you didn't know how old you were?" Too many people would say they feel or look older than they are. If that is the case, you can change it.

Aging is inevitable. The pace at which we're pulled along in life, however, can be influenced. I'm not referring to any "anti-aging" remedy—a popular myth connected with many dietary supplements, drugs, and diets. We can influence aging by creating a body that functions physiologically younger than our chronological age. *This* is real.

Chronological age refers to how young or old we are measured on the calendar; physiological age refers to how well, or poor, we function. Those with few risk factors for chronic disease, for example, and with good fitness, may be considered physiologically younger than someone the same age who is unhealthy.

When comparing a person's physiology with their calendar age, we find some are healthier and more fit—in other words, relatively younger and more vibrant than their age in years. All the issues addressed in this book relate to improving one's physiological age.

Although scientists continue to probe the questions about why and what makes some older athletes so great, the general answer is quite clear: the process begins by being both healthy and fit.

Over the Hill?

Most people start focusing more on aging sometime around their thirtieth birthday. At this stage of life, maximal oxygen uptake (VO_{2max}) begins a steady decline, diminishing 5 to 15 percent each decade. Likewise for the maximum heart rate, with the average person losing six to ten beats every ten years. These changes are due in great part from reductions in cardiac output. This is the amount of blood that pumps out of the heart each minute. Along with other changes in the cardiovascular system, including those in the heart itself, the result is less blood—and therefore oxygen and nutrients— reaching the muscles. Part of this decline also includes a reduction in the lung's capacity to take in oxygen and expel carbon dioxide.

By remaining fit and healthy, however, one can slow the pace of these declines. For example, a balanced athlete may reduce the decline of VO_{2max} by half.

Those who better control the decline have certain profiles:

- They avoid excess body fat. It's particularly important to evade too much belly fat because it's association with carbohydrate intolerance, which also increases with age and comes with the risk of cardiovascular disease.
- Carbohydrate intolerance means we don't get away with eating sugar, white flour, cereals, and desserts like we used to. In many cases, we are not able to eat natural carbohydrates as much, either—beans, rice, fruits, and others sometimes considered healthy. When consuming more carbs than we should, our

energy suffers, blood pressure rises, blood fats elevate, and other problems develop.

- Muscle mass can also decline with age, and this too can be offset with good health, especially a great diet with adequate protein. Otherwise, the double-trouble of dropping muscle and increasing body fat could actually depress VO_{2max} faster, not to mention impair overall health.

- In addition, maintaining hormone balance is vital to offset the pace of aging. One common problem may be associated with the stress hormone cortisol. When physical, chemical, and mental stressors, such as overtraining and poor diet, are not well regulated, cortisol rises causing the production of sex hormones to crash. In particular, testosterone and the estrogens, in both men and women, are necessary to maintain an athlete's health and fitness well into the upper age groups.

- Other physical factors become noticeable with aging. Quickness has already reduced itself in noticeable ways, as has natural flexibility.

But athletes heading into their forties, fifties, sixties, and beyond have something to cheer about.

The Good News

Factors such as VO_{2max} and maximum heart rate are associated with more intense anaerobic activities. Even the loss of muscle can be misleading—the fibers that are lost are mostly the anaerobic ones, the reason we lose quick reaction and sprint speed. Endurance training, on the other hand, is performed at sub-max levels, relying on slow-twitch aerobic muscles. This system helps the body compensation for the diminished cardiovascular function and the ability of the body to deliver oxygen to muscles. It means we can still improve our endurance at any age.

Consider too that most races lasting two or three hours are performed closer to the sub-max state—and those with better fat burning will compete better. The ability to burn more fats for energy is not impaired in the healthy aging athlete—one reason so many excel beyond the performances of the fellow athletes twenty or more years younger. That is, unless one allows carbohydrate intolerance to develop, reducing the ability to burn more fat for the aerobic system.

Many of today's athletes find ways to ward off progressing age, remaining physiologically younger. Overall, runners in their sixties and seventies have surpassed the winning times for sprints and the marathon at the first Olympic Games of 1896. If that does not impress everyone, consider some of these amazing feats by "older" elite athletes:

- Meb Keflezighi was one month shy of turning 39 when he won the 2014 Boston Marathon.
- At age 41, Dara Torres became the oldest swimmer on the U.S. Olympic team. She won three silver medals in the 2008 Games.
- Ethiopia's Haile Gebrselassie was thirty-five when he set a marathon world record of 2:03:59 in 2008.
- Priscilla Welch was the first women finisher in the 1987 New York City Marathon at age forty-two. (Earlier that year she was second in the London Marathon with a time of 2:26:51.)
- Mark Allen won the last of his six Ironman World Championships in 1996 at age thirty-eight.
- Portugal's Carlos Lopes was thirty-seven when he won the 1984 Los Angeles Olympic marathon. At age thirty-eight he won the Rotterdam Marathon in 2:07:12, breaking the world record by nearly a minute.

Also, consider these other amazing efforts:

- In 2014, Harriette Thompson, ninety-one, finished the Rock 'n' Roll San Diego Marathon in 7:07:42 (a record for her age group).

- In 2011, Fauja Singh, a one-hundred-year-old runner became the world's oldest person to complete a marathon: 8:25:16 at the Scotiabank Toronto Waterfront race.
- In 2011, Lew Hollander, eighty-one, became the oldest Ironman finisher at the World Championships in Kona, Hawaii, beating eighty-one-year-old France Cokan.
- In 2003, Canadian Ed Whitlock became the oldest person at age seventy-three to run a marathon in under three hours.

What is clear with these and many other achievements by those in their forties and above is that human endurance does not decline like our anaerobic, power systems. In addition, many of us have experienced other examples of physiologically younger yet chronologically older athletes passing us during a race. It's not unusual to see athletes higher up in age groups finish events far ahead of many other competitors in younger age categories.

If there is a problem with athletes who reach fifty, sixty, and beyond, it's reduced health. Whether it's a lifetime of injuries, poor diet, or undue stress, the wear and tear is evident in many. This, along with medication, is a reason that aerobic training needs to proceed at lower-than-desired heart rates.

The 180 Penalty?

One of the very common questions I receive has to do with training heart rates and why many athletes have to initially slow down using the 180 formula. This is particularly true when it comes from those in their fifties, sixties, and above. "It's like a penalty," one sixty-six-year-old athlete commented.

There is really no age penalty in the 180 formula. It does depend in part on both physiological and chronological age, as the four options in the formula demonstrate.

For another perspective, consider that VO_{2max} and maximum heart rates diminish significantly over one's lifespan. Even the 220 formulas, even though they are very inaccurate, lead to lower rates for seniors. So it would make sense that the 180 formula training heart rate would have a corresponding lower rate, especially if you relate it to those obtained by younger athletes.

Here's an important fact: Athletes of all ages, including those in the fifties, sixties, seventies, and above age group can still improve endurance, sometimes significantly. This means proper training, supported by a great diet, will lead to faster MAF tests and better race performance.

The only real penalty we may be given when using the 180 formula is for not being as healthy as possible. Athletes of all ages are penalized when they have frequent colds or other illness, allergies or asthma, or other conditions. This is particularly true for those taking medications—an indication of a significant health problem, most of which are preventable. While this brings the training heart rate down ten big beats, with improved training and lifestyle, eliminating medication is a real possibility. There is also a caveat in the Formula that allows for an addition of ten beats for those who are very healthy. This is what you can do after making lifestyle changes that significantly improve health.

Preparticipation Screening

It's unfortunate that there are too few health practitioners who can truly help you reach your health and fitness goals. However, there are many who can screen you for disease, thus possibly saving your life. Here are three important points in this process.

1. Oral History—Critical Questions

By far the most important feature of an evaluation by a health practitioner is a detailed history—getting to know you face-to-face is vital. Of course, this cannot be accomplished when the time spent in an initial evaluation is too few minutes. Along with finding a practitioner who is also an athlete, one willing to spend adequate time taking your history is most important.

Here are some of the key questions to help rule out serious conditions:

- Chest pain or discomfort?
- Shortness of breath?
- Unexpected fatigue?
- History of heart murmur?
- High blood pressure?
- Family history of heart disease or premature death?

2. Physical Examination

After a complete history, an examination follows. The extent of it can vary with the individual's history. It probably includes listening to your heart and lungs, taking blood pressure, and other common evaluations. But an electrocariogram (EKG), blood, urine, and other tests depend on your history and exam findings.

3. Stress Test.

While exercise stress testing has not been shown to be cost effective in large screening programs of younger athletes, it is appropriate in the older athlete under three conditions:

- With known cardiovascular disease.
- When cardiovascular symptoms suggest it.
- When risk factors are present, including hypertension and diabetes.

While the American College of Sports Medicine recommends exercise stress testing in men older than forty years and women older than fifty years before starting a vigorous exercise program, your health practitioner, who knows you best, should make these and other important recommendations.

4. Some Reasons to Avoid Training and Racing.

- Active myocarditis or pericarditis (inflammation of the heart).
- Suspected coronary artery disease or other conditions, including abnormal EKG.
- Uncontrolled hypertension (high blood pressure).
- Recent history of concussion.
- Physical damage to muscle, joint, or other body area.

Training on Meds: Adjusting the Heart Rate

People are so surprised when my response to their question "What medications are you taking?" is a flat *none*. Whether in a dental office or a blood lab, the reactions still surprise me. They often have a follow up, such as "which over-the-counter meds do you take?" *None* is the answer again. Sometimes, the person uses my answer to repeat the question, as if my hearing is bad, which it is not: "No meds?" *No*.

The problem, of course, is that many people are on meds, including athletes. Nearly 70 percent of Americans are on at least one prescription drug, and more than half take two, Mayo Clinic researchers say. Twenty percent of patients are on five or more prescriptions, and, of course, too many take more.

Prescription drug use increases with age, with more that 88 percent of those over age sixty taking at least one medication, while a distressing 36 percent of this age group takes five or more different prescription drugs.

In addition, up to 50 percent of people may be using over-the-counter medications. While many of these medicines were once prescription-only, they all have the real potential for side effects, and, with two or more, adverse drug interactions.

Many Drugs Affect Heart Rate

For athletes on medication, reducing the training heart rate by an additional ten beats is a hard pill to swallow. But the math is actually quite straightforward, with the Formula containing this caveat:

If you are taking any regular medication, subtract ten. Not only is this relevant to prescription and over-the-counter drugs that modify your heart rate during exercise, it applies to *any* medication. The result is a further lowering of the aerobic training heart rate, slowing the intensity of the workout, at least for the moment. It's always best to be conservative and always a good idea to ask your doctor about medication, training, and racing.

While some may think prescription and over-the-counter drugs are all perfectly safe, or that the health problems associated with their needs are quite innocuous, this is absolutely not the case most of the time. So being more conservative during exercise is important to prevent problems of excessive stress or overtraining from your workouts. There's still a wide range of intensity below the maximum aerobic heart rate that will provide significant benefits. In addition, this will help with optimal development of the aerobic system often to the point at which your doctor may reduce a drug's dosage, or decide the medication is no longer necessary.

A second reason to subtract ten beats in the 180 formula for a person on any regular medication has to do with overall health. The fact that a healthcare professional has prescribed or recommended a drug means that you have some significant health problem.

Even though many medications don't directly affect the heart rate, the impact on health can adversely affect muscles, metabolism, and other systems of the body that promote health and fitness. An example includes a group of cholesterol-lowering drugs called *statins*, including Mevacor, Lipator, and Altocor, the most commonly prescribed drugs. These can affect muscle function, sometimes leading to exercise-related injuries. By making the ten-beat adjustment in heart rate, the risk of muscle problems and potential injuries may be reduced.

Another example is aspirin and other NSAIDs, which can interfere with proper recovery after exercise. By working out at a lower heart rate, the stress on the physical body will be reduced along with better recovery.

Even for a woman who is taking birth control pills or hormone replacement therapy, these medications have potential side effects that can adversely affect exercise activity. In this case, the levels of some B vitamins can be lowered, affecting liver function, energy systems, lactate production, and other important body functions necessary for optimal health and fitness.

For athletes, training at a lower heart rate may result in slower progress, but getting faster at that same rate and improvements in performances should still be realized.

Are meds really needed?

I am not opposed to the use of medications—but I am opposed to how they are prescribed. Sometimes this is performed properly, matching the patient's condition with a particular drug. Too often, however, prescriptions are handed out irresponsibly, and too often patients accumulate too many meds.

It's very possible that by improving health, including eliminating junk food, and developing the aerobic system, the need for medication may disappear.

A note on caffeine: I don't recommend making further adjustments in the 180 formula for those drinking small or modest amounts of coffee before working out. Clearly, this can affect the heart rate. But like eating a bowl of junk-food cereal or a bagel, which can adversely affect endurance performance by reducing fat burning, I choose not to adjust the training heart rate for these habits.

Keys to Successful Aging

Virtually all mammals on earth have a lifespan six times their skeletal maturity. If we apply this animal model to humans, who reach skeletal maturity at about age twenty, one should expect to live, on average, to age 120. In fact, scientists have isolated the genetic blueprints that allow us to live into our hundreds. Following our understanding of gene expression, it may simply be that most individuals don't allow that particular gene to keep them alive because diet, exercise, stress, and other factors impair the genetic process.

In our society, the average human animal barely reaches four times his or her skeletal maturity. According to the U.S. Census Bureau, only about twenty-three out of each 100,000 people reach birthday number one hundred. But with modern technology, natural hygiene, and the awareness of chemicals that speed the aging process, there will soon be hundreds of thousands of people in the United States over the age of one hundred. The Bureau estimates that by 2050 there will be between 265,000 and possibly four million centenarians.

Will you be one of them? And if so, will you welcome it, considering what your quality of life might be? While there is a genetic aspect to how long you will live, there also are many lifestyle factors that may be even more important. How well you care for yourself from the earliest age has a significant impact on both the length and quality of your life.

Unfortunately, most people don't think they'll live that long, and many actually hope they won't. However, others welcome the challenge and excitement of seeing a fifth-generation descendant running his or her first road race.

But who wants to watch this celebrated event in a wheelchair, unaware of where you are, what the name of the descendant is, or who his or her parents are? If you do happen to live to one hundred—or 120 years young—you want to be fully functional. You might even want to run that race too.

The term "successful" or "healthy" aging is not a catchy phrase or new program. It's a real concept with practical applications for people of all ages. Scientists note three common paths for people as they age.

- "Successful aging" results in a higher quality of life.
- "Usual aging" would be considered "average."
- Finally, "diseased aging" results in low quality of life and slow death.

Average is unacceptable, and diseased is no way to live or to die. The better you age, the higher your quality of life, the more productive you are throughout life, and the less likely you will die a slow, lingering death.

The younger you are, physiologically, the more you can do to control how well you age. The older you are, the more you want to control aging. Regardless of your age now, your current actions can have significant impact on the way you age.

Seven Factors For Healthy Aging

In my years of practice and research I have identified several key factors that can have a direct and powerful impact on how successfully we age. These are among the habits I strictly follow. As you read this list, you'll notice it's a review of many concepts that I have put forth throughout my career.

1. Brain nutrients and brain stimulation
2. Anti-inflammatory foods
3. Antioxidant foods
4. Avoiding refined carbohydrates and sugars (junk food)
5. Eating adequate protein foods
6. Building aerobic fitness
7. Controlling stress

Successful aging also includes the issues involving a person's need to love, have fun, to socialize, and feel good about life. While volumes have been written about these topics and their effects on aging, my contention is that when people take the necessary steps to better health, they feel better mentally and emotionally, and tend to socialize and enjoy life more, which leads to better overall mental health.

Lynn Peters Adler, a former lawyer who founded and runs the National Centenarian Awareness Project, has been working with centenarians for twenty-five years, and sees certain similarities among them, including:

- A positive but realistic attitude
- A love of life
- A sense of humor
- Spirituality
- Courage

A remarkable ability to accept the losses that come with age but not be stopped by them.

Aging Posture and Gait

We can all update our age, and always strive to be younger. While we know that most debilitating chronic illnesses are preventable, including heart disease, cancer, and Alzheimer's, so is poor aging. Large numbers of today's elderly are living longer through heroic measures such as heart, lung, and liver transplants, around the clock care and other medical means. For most, those "extra years" come at the end of the lifespan, unfortunately, when life is less vigorous and productive. But we can significantly control what may be the most important factor of aging—quality of life. And the sooner we start the better.

While the whole body plays a role in graceful aging, three areas in particular do much of the work:

- The brain-muscle mechanism
- Hormones
- The immune system

These areas of the body are continuously repairing and replacing themselves, relying on raw materials from the foods we eat. Adelle Davis's 1950s mantra, "you are what you eat," still holds true today.

These and other aging factors are so integrated into our whole body that it is difficult to discuss each one in isolation. For example, hormones are an essential part of immunity, and muscle function reflects physical, chemical, and mental health. In particular, two of the most common images of aging—posture and gait—are also signs of how well we are doing it.

The Bent Spine Syndrome

Among the most common images of poor aging are people who do not stand erect. On closer examination, they don't sit or move that way either, especially when walking. Their lower (lumbar) spine is flexed, and they are "bent" forward having lost their natural spinal curve, which usually helps maintain a healthy-looking upright posture. With a "bent" spine, individuals become shorter. While this is most noticeable in the elderly, the process sometimes begins in the younger years. This condition is well recognized by clinicians and researchers, and is called the *bent spine syndrome*, BSS, originally referred to as camptocormia, derived from the Greek camptos (bent) and kormos (trunk).

The BSS is a spectrum disorder, going from mild and moderate to a more severe condition depending on a person's level of health. Two common causes of BSS include muscle imbalances, often a reflection of various neurological and biochemical problems, and psychological disorders.

The BSS effects the whole body, not just the spine. An example is how proper spinal function can help balance a key component of the body, the autonomic nervous system, which regulates many aspects of health from blood pressure, heartbeat, and breathing, to gut function, sexual arousal, and controlling all stress.

As a functional problem for most individuals, BSS is rarely due to permanent changes in the bones or discs of the spinal column. This is evident when lying down—in this relaxed position people with BSS have relatively straight spines.

In addition, BSS may or may not be associated with pain, but it always causes stress. The posture and gait are typically irregular, with related body-wide function that can be significantly reduced. The result is poor aging.

Physical and Chemical Causes

There are a number of physical causes of BSS, perhaps the most common one being muscle imbalance (muscles directly control the skeleton, especially the spine). In most cases, these imbalances are due to some type of neurological dysfunction between the brain and muscle. These weaknesses are not only in muscles directly controlling the spine, but throughout the body, too, including those in the feet, pelvis, abdomen, and neck—areas that can significantly affect spinal posture and movement.

Another aspect of muscle dysfunction is reduced energy due to chemical imbalance. Muscle fatigue develops quickly in those with BSS during standing, walking, and even easy physical activities. This is typically due to poor aerobic metabolism.

Other biochemical factors include abnormally high levels of fat found in the muscles of those with BSS. The cause of this may be of hormonal, primarily high insulin due to the ingestion of too much refined carbohydrate. Higher levels of the stress hormone cortisol also can influence the brain, often significantly. This is typically due to the combination of physical, chemical, and mental stressors, which, in turn, can effect muscle balance.

At any age, BSS is associated with—often caused by—other chemical disorders that include chronic inflammation. This is usually directly associated with the balance of fat in the diet. The ongoing inflammatory disorder is the first stage of many chronic diseases.

Other hormonal imbalance can play a role, too. Particularly important are conditions of low testosterone and low thyroid function—both can occur in men and women. In addition, low levels of vitamin D, typically from inadequate sun exposure, and sarcopenia, the loss of muscle during aging, are both very common problems of epidemic proportion that can speed up the aging process.

More severe cases of BSS are often seen in patients with Parkinson's disease, multiple sclerosis, or other neurological diseases.

Psychology

It has long been known that posture and gait, in addition to being a manifestation of physical and chemical dysfunction affecting muscle contraction, can also reflect one's psychological state. Bent spine syndrome was first observed and researched in young soldiers psychologically affected by war. Whether old or young, images of an aging spine can reflect mental and emotional states.

Growing Younger

Just being aware of ones posture is the first step to improved function. By avoiding the common age- or fatigue-related slumping and making sure the lower spine is not slowly losing its natural curve, one can keep the body healthier and not only more youthful looking, but physiologically younger. By simply sitting up straight, standing, walking, and running more erect, we can maintain better balance, and our bodies will function better.

In addition, yoga, tai chi, respiratory biofeedback, and other self-therapies can be very effective in maintaining good posture when practiced properly.

Regardless of how much or little you run, bike, or lift weights, walking can also do wonders to help train the brain to better maintain proper postures. Walking erect is part of an optimal walking gait. In order to do this effectively, the knees must be gently locked as you land more on the front of your heels. This is different from the running (or jogging) gait, where knees should never lock and landing on the foot is farther forward. (By striking on the back of the heels, often encouraged by wearing thicker shoes, many runners do lock their knees, which can directly cause knee and other physical impairments, poor gait, and wasted energy.)

While most of us are too familiar with the images of aging, we sometimes don't see it in ourselves. We can control the process significantly.

Is Aging a Disease?

Should aging be viewed as a disease that can be treated or delayed? This question may sound rather odd, but there are many scientists who have been addressing it for years, and most answer with a definitive "yes." This same question is the title of a published editorial in the journal *Frontiers in Aging Neuroscience* (2011) by Dr. Ruth Elaine Nieuwenhuis-Mark of the Department of Medical Psychology and Neuropsychology at Tilburg University, the Netherlands.

This groundswell of support for calling aging a disease is undergoing the process of re-educating both the public and health authorities. Many research specialists in aging are lobbying the world's biggest drug regulator, the U.S. Food and Drug Administration, to consider defining the process of aging as a disease. This will most likely take place because it has already happened with other "conditions" such as obesity, a preventable lifestyle problem and not a disease in the real sense of the word.

By considering aging a disease, researchers are making the claim that it can be "treated" and delayed. Most importantly, branding age as a disease would speed the development of new drugs that treat many of the "effects" of aging—including diabetes, cancer, heart disease, and Alzheimer's. Currently, scientists argue that they are being hampered in their efforts by the FDA, who approves drugs only for specific diseases, not for something as general, natural, or normal as aging.

Do we really need a whole new line of drugs that attempts to increase longevity?

Dr. Nieuwenhuis-Mark's editorial concludes by claiming that making the jump to call aging a disease is, "at the very least, questionable, and indeed, worrisome." She asks, "Do we really need to feed the already negative stereotypes which exist of the elderly in society? Should we not be celebrating how much the old bring to the world and have still to offer not only to close family and friends but also to society at large?" She closes with, "Labeling aging as a disease may or may not help research funding but it can only hurt public opinion of what it means to age."

Muscle Loss and Aging

To maintain optimal endurance for training and racing, muscles are obviously an important factor. While muscle loss is common, it is something we can avoid.

Muscle atrophy appears to result from a gradual loss of both muscle fiber size and number. Reductions in the muscle's cross-sectional area is often found with advancing age; by age fifty, about 10 percent of muscle area is gone. After fifty years of age, the rate of accelerates significantly. Muscle strength declines by approximately 15 percent per decade in the sixties and seventies and by about 30 percent thereafter.

But a variety of health and fitness factors can reduce, and perhaps even stop the decline. Sure we won't be able to bench press the same heavy weights we did at age thirty, but sufficient strength and mass can be saved. One key factor is the need to consume adequate protein. Please take the health survey below.

Do You Have Any of the Problems Listed Below?

1. Reduced muscle strength
2. Muscle imbalance (aches and pains, chronic injuries)
3. Hormone imbalance
4. Carbohydrate intolerance
5. Chronic inflammation
6. Reduced physical performance
7. Poor balance
8. Low vitamin D (blood test below 50 nmol/L)
9. Eat meat, fish, or eggs less than three times a day
10. Taking antacids or drugs to reduce stomach acid

These are common signs and symptoms associated with chronic protein malnutrition. Even one or two of these items may indicate you're losing muscle.

Protein Foods

The image many people have of protein foods is that they're mostly for body builders, weight lifters, and football players. The fact is everyone needs daily dietary protein to be healthy and fit. We require it to meet our basic nutritional requirements to help build and maintain our bones, organs, and glands. We use dietary protein to make health-promoting enzymes for energy, hormone balance, digestion, and immune function. And, protein is very important for the brain.

We also need to consume protein each day to replace the millions of muscle cells we normally lose. Otherwise, muscle mass can diminish. By maintaining them, we not only sustain our strength and ability to be agile, we also protect our bones, and prevent injury.

At one time low muscle mass was considered a problem mostly in those over age sixty, but now it's a health issue in younger adults and even children. Why? The overfat epidemic—more people are getting overfat with less muscle. Lower levels of muscle are significantly associated carbohydrate intolerance and chronic inflammation.

What is Sarcopenia?

Many people complain about getting old. They slow down, have more aches and pains, and lose strength. Their balance is lost, risking falls and broken bones. I'm not only talking about seventy- and eighty-year-olds, but even people in their forties and fifties have these signs and symptoms. In time, the slow reduction in height, and poor posture, which may have begun years earlier, becomes evident. The problem is sarcopenia—the loss of muscle that typically accompanies the ageing process. A key cause is inadequate dietary protein intake. It's also a major cause of physical disability, loss of independence, and frailty.

In the September 7, 2010, issue of the medical journal *Clinical Interventions in Aging* ("Optimal Management of Sarcopenia"), researchers Louise Burton and Deepa Sumukadas from University of Dundee in Scotland write that, "Many older adults do not consume sufficient amounts of dietary protein which leads to a reduction in lean body mass and increased functional impairment." They also explain that the loss of muscle mass is a strong predictor of mortality in later life, and that low strength, the result of lost muscle, is associated with increased risk of death.

Our muscle mass peaks in our twenties and thirties, and by our forties starts to drop. By fifty there is a steady decline in our muscles throughout the body. But it need not be the case in everyone—we control much of these changes through lifestyle.

One main reason we lose muscle is from reduced intake of protein (the other has to do with low levels of physical activity). Just eating sufficient amounts of protein foods not only can help maintain muscle mass, but also prevent sarcopenia.

But the problem of low muscle mass is no longer just one of aging. Even young people, including children, are not building their bodies early in life. Preethi Srikanthan and colleagues from UCLA's Department of Medicine write in a May 2010 issue of the medical journal *PLOS*, "With the ongoing obesity epidemic in the U.S. and the disturbing increases in the incidence of obesity in children and young adults, our data suggest that we can expect to see sharp increases in sarcopenia and diabetes in the coming years. In this environment, interventions aimed at increasing muscle mass in younger ages and preventing loss of muscle mass in older ages may have the potential to reduce type 2 diabetes risk."

Because muscles do more than move our bodies (see Section 6), lowered muscle mass can also cause poor circulation, reduced immune function, especially in controlling free radicals, and can place us at risk for carbohydrate intolerance and diabetes, increased blood fats (cholesterol and triglycerides), hypertension, and cardiovascular disease.

As body function diminishes and ill health rises, sarcopenia can worsen to a more advanced condition called cachexia—a metabolic syndrome with chronic inflammation at its root, with even more loss of the body's muscles. Where sarcopenia ends and cachexia begins is difficult to distinguish, but the key is preventing both by maintaining optimal protein intake and physical activity.

Coming Soon: The Sarcopenia Scan Scam

Like the rage in bone scans in recent decades, scanning the body's muscle mass will soon become the latest healthcare trend. It will be done not to inform you to eat better and encourage better workouts, but to sell you some special dietary supplement or "new" workout DVD specifically designed for muscle loss. New drugs will also become popular. But none of these will be better than just eating right, including protein every day, and balanced training.

Two accurate methods of measuring muscle mass is magnetic resonance imaging (MRI), considered to be the most accurate, and dual energy X-ray absorptiometry (DXA) as it also measures both fat and bone mass. They are not perfect as the tests are difficult in distinguishing muscle from water retention, and muscle fat. Bioelectric Impedence Analysis is a cheaper, quicker, noninvasive method for measuring muscle, but its reliability varies with an individual's hydration status, ethnicity, physical fitness, and age.

How much protein?

The answer to this question depends on you and your particular needs. Factors such as lean body mass (how much muscle you have), your level of physical activity, and what makes you feel best after a meal, can help guide you. There is a wide range of healthy protein intake. General estimates on protein needs can be made by a percent of calories in your diet, or, with a more detailed approach using a range of normal using the USDA's guidelines as the bare minimum needs.

While triathletes, cyclists, and other endurance athletes usually have noticeable amounts of muscle mass, marathoners seem to have very little. This is deceiving. A full 40 percent of an endurance male athlete's body weight may be muscle, less in women. Training results in a daily turnover of muscle that needs repair and replacement, which can be significant. How much dietary protein does this require? It varies with the individual. But because body weight is related to one's muscle mass, the following can be used as a guide.

Minimum daily protein needs may be about 1.6 grams of protein per kilogram of body weight, or about 3.5 grams per pound. Let's put this into sharper perspective in terms of servings of protein foods:

- For a 145-pound athlete, the requirement may be about 106 grams. This can be obtained from two eggs for breakfast, a chef's salad for lunch, and a small sirloin steak for dinner.
- An athlete weighing 125 pounds would minimally require about ninety grams of protein. This can be obtained from two eggs at breakfast, fish for lunch, and lamb for dinner.

You can adjust the exact proportion to your own weight. By sticking to these general guidelines, athletes can learn that a diet comprised of 30 percent protein might be about right.

Why Animal Protein is Essential

The human intestinal track is well adapted for digesting animal-source foods, having evolved on a diet that included meat and fish (with varying amounts of vegetables, fruits, seeds, and nuts). While the popular trend in recent decades has been toward the misconception that meat consumption is unhealthy—and this may be true if they are not healthy and well cared for, and organic—there are a variety of unique features of an animal-food diet that are vital for health and fitness. Here are some of them:

- Animal foods contain high levels of all essential amino acids.
- Vitamin B12 is an essential nutrient found only in animal foods.

- EPA, the powerful omega-3 fat that helps control inflammation, and the one preferred by the human body, is almost exclusively found in animal foods.
- Iron deficiency is a common worldwide problem and is best prevented by eating animal food because it contains this mineral in a most bioavailable form.
- Vitamin A is found only in animal products. Vegetables and fruits contain beta carotene which is not vitamin A; its conversion in the body to vitamin A is not always efficient in humans.
- Animal products are dense protein foods with little or no carbohydrate to interfere with digestion and absorption.
- People who consume less animal protein have greater rates of bone loss than those who eat larger amounts of animal protein.
- Creatine, the best source is meat, is an important amino acid to build muscle and prevent its loss.
- The amino acid glutamine, the main energy source for optimal intestinal function, is primarily found in meat, especially those minimally cooked such as rare beef.

Preventing loss of muscle mass with aging, and building and maintaining muscles in people of all ages is vital for optimal health and fitness. Eating sufficient protein every day, along with balanced physical activity, accomplishes this task quite easily.

Making Changes

If your body and brain are not the best they can be, change them. As you go through this book, and especially the other Big books, you will easily see topics important for you to work on. Let's use the issue of hypertension as an example.

High blood pressure is a common and dangerous condition. In the U.S., about a third of adults have high blood pressure, with more than half of them either unaware of it or it is uncontrolled. Also called hypertension, it increases the risk for heart disease and stroke, two leading causes of death. Aging itself is considered a risk factor for high blood pressure. The CDC reports that nine out of ten Americans will develop hypertension during their life. Other countries have similar sad statistics. But this is just the tip of the iceberg.

Among the problems that may contribute to hypertension is carbohydrate intolerance due to its influence of raising insulin levels. During the Two-Week Test it was recommended that, if your blood pressure is high, have it evaluated before, during, and after the Test. That's because for many people, significantly reducing refined carbohydrates and sugars, which reduces insulin levels, will lower blood pressure—often dramatically. As a result, if you're taking medication to control blood pressure, your doctor may need to reduce, or even eliminate it.

The vast majority of hypertensive patients I initially saw in practice were able to reduce their blood pressure significantly just by strictly avoiding refined carbohydrates and sugars, especially when developing the aerobic system was implemented. Most of these patients were able to eliminate their medication. Other important factors include balancing fats, various nutrients that can be obtained from a healthy diet, and controlling stress.

Poor aerobic conditioning can contribute to hypertension. Recall that those who are inactive have a significant amount of blood vessels shut down (these are the vessels in the aerobic muscle fibers). Aerobic exercise is an important factor in both prevention and treatment of hypertension. Even one easy aerobic workout can reduce blood pressure for up to twenty-four hours. Anaerobic exercise may not be nearly as effective and could even aggravate high blood pressure. It's important to discuss your particular exercise needs with a healthcare professional—especially one who is an athlete, and aware of the potential benefits of healthy food.

But the problem is not just about hypertension. It's not only about being at high risk for heart disease, or being depressed. Whatever signs and symptoms led to the need for medication, there's a good chance you can change it—if you're successful, you can go back to the 180 formula and modify it by adding back ten beats.

Adding "10" to Your Training Heart Rate

While many athletes following the 180 formula would like to train at higher heart rates, too many other health and fitness factors don't allow it. But you can change that. Once you make significant lifestyle modifications that bring better and stable body function, simply go back to re-work the formula again.

Here are two case histories:

- Joseph was having difficulty training slow. While his chronic injuries had finally disappeared, he missed running fast with his friends. But medication for high blood pressure was necessary. Desperate to improve his racing, Joseph finally agreed to take the Two-Week Test and eliminate all junk foods, along with moderate and high glycemic natural carbohydrates. He felt great after the test, with about a thirty second per mile improvement in his MAF Test. And his blood pressure reduced significantly. This made Joseph excited enough to remain on the same eating routine as during the Two-Week Test. I suggested returning to his cardiologist for a re-evaluation, which he did two weeks later. Joseph was even more excited to find out that his blood pressure was getting too low, and, after some experimentation, his doctor said he no longer needed medication. After another month, with stable blood pressure, I recommended Joseph add ten beats to his training heart rate. Five months later, Joseph ran his best marathon in 2:58—a personal best by more than nineteen minutes.
- Irene struggled with her weight for many years despite being very active as an open water swimmer. At age fifty she decided to start running, and a year later added cycling. Competing in a triathlon as a goal, her training heart rate had been adjusted down because she took two different medications for her high

blood cholesterol and triglycerides. While she struggled with carbohydrate addiction, she was determined to race better in the next age group now only two years away. Finally, through *cold turkey*, she stopped eating all sugar and refined carbohydrates. A month later her MAF Test showed the first improvement in over two years. I recommended a blood test, but she wanted to wait. For the next three months her cycling and running got faster. She finally checked her blood, and both cholesterol and triglycerides were normal. Without medication, we added ten beats to her training heart rate. She almost immediately complained that cycling was too fast and it was difficult to maintain her training heart rate. With the addition of aerobic intervals, and a continual improvement in aerobic running speed, Irene easily won her age group at a large triathlon.

Of course, it's not always possible to eliminate medication. But by significantly improving health and fitness, many can accomplish this feat.

You can manipulate aging as much as you can influence disease prevention and most other factors associated with health and fitness. It's less about the information—there's enough in this book to keep you busy for some time—and more about another important factor: taking action. The first step in this whole process is entirely in your hands. You decide to increase your athleticism, or, often through *inaction*, decide not to pursue it. Yet it's my hope that you follow through on the affirmative. It's never too late to make important lifestyle and dietary changes. And once that decision is made, you will happily discover that you have only just begun the exciting journey through the rest of your life.

FIT BUT UNHEALTHY

The story of the ancient Greek runner Pheidippides inspired the modern day marathon. He is known for dying after a long run to declare a battle's victory. Some of my boyhood memories are of great athletes unexpectedly dying. It was difficult to grasp how heroes could suddenly drop dead. Ultimately, the study of human physiology brought the answer: they were remarkable fit, but unhealthy. Despite certain advances in healthcare, this unfortunate problem continues today as more endurance athletes train harder and longer, and eat unnatural food.

The athletic world is full of the apparent paradox of athletes who are fit enough to perform great feats, but at the same time have low levels of health, rendering them vulnerable to injury, illness, disease, and sometimes death.

Athletes: Fit but Unhealthy

For a long time, researchers have been looking at how the high demands of endurance training and racing can increase the risk of death. Dr. John Mandrola's Medscape review of a new study in the *European Heart Journal* sums it up this way: "The idea that long-term endurance exercise increases the risk for arrhythmia should no longer be considered counterintuitive. The list of published studies confirming this association is long, and this week, it got a little longer." This new study looked at abnormal heart conditions (specifically, potentially deadly arrhythmias), showing poor cardiac health in a group of more than fifty thousand high-level endurance athletes—the most fit were more likely to have heart problems.

But there is a real problem with these studies. The media coverage misses it too. It is not in the subjects chosen or with other research protocol. A primary issue is almost never addressed—the big picture. Sure, it is a sensitive subject. The idea that a dedicated, hard working, young athlete is hurting his or her heart is shattering to the image of a social icon. We unfortunately accept knee injuries, hip pain, and tendon tears, even in a non-contact sport—but death? That shatters the legends of athletes who are held at such high esteem. What is missing is the idea that these serious conditions are not part of a healthy body, and almost all are preventable.

Fitness is the ability to be athletic. Health is different, being a state where all the body's systems are working in harmony. While one can exist without the other, athletes who are healthy have lower rates of injury, whether in the knee or heart, have longer and more successful careers, and better quality of life in later years. Those with reduced health can suffer consequences. This comes in some form of physical, chemical, and or mental stress.

John Lennon wrote, "There's room at the top they are telling you still; but first you must learn how to smile as you kill." We live in a cutthroat world, one of "no pain, no gain" at seemingly every level. "More is better" is a modern mantra. It is no surprise that this mentality is mirrored in sports, and not just on the professional levels, but for the many millions of joggers, serious runners and cyclists, triathletes, and other endurance athletes. More miles, more speed, more racing, more carbs—just do it. And if that doesn't get us to the top (of the pack, our age group, our personal goals), we train harder. Then, there is the option of doping.

Like the over-stressed, out-of-shape Wall Street executive who dies at his desk of a heart attack at age forty, athletes are not immune to premature, preventable death either, from the same cause. This is an unfortunate fact. In a world where war is celebrated, warriors of all types are placed on the edge of high pedestals.

The full spectrum of health problems can occur in endurance athletes of all types, and in every age group and both genders. And virtually all can be avoided.

There are some common underlying conditions in athletes who develop heart disease:

- Overtraining can play a dominant role in causing significant stress. This includes too much training volume and or intensity. Even the American Heart Association's guidelines for physical activity cautions against too much high intensity training.
- Chronic inflammation is associated with both overtraining and poor diet. Both can contribute to heart disease.
- The overconsumption of refined carbohydrates can contribute to chronic inflammation, increased body fat, and is commonly associated with the overtraining syndrome.

Not surprisingly, the above conditions typically precede many common injuries of muscles, joints, ligaments, and other breakdowns.

Perhaps the most important point is that if you're an endurance athlete, frequent high volume and intense training is not necessary to reach one's potential. Whether it is winning the Ironman, an age group, or just completing a particular endurance event, balanced workouts can bring success. Eating well is a vital part of the plan.

Unhealthy Olympians: Who is to Blame?

Since the release of *The Big Book of Endurance Training and Racing*, there has been another Summer Olympic Games. And once again stories about fit but unhealthy athletes were everywhere.

The lead story in *Sports Illustrated* online began, "Almost every dominant performance in London has raised eyebrows, if not questions. These are today's Olympics." While the article went on to discuss the unhealthy issue of doping in sports, those two simple sentences brought to mind an even more serious and greater common problem.

Hundreds of millions of people around the world watched the London 2012 Olympic Games on TV. They saw some great performances, heart-breaking disappointments, and a lot of advertising for junk food.

Certainly, junk food has contributed not only to the worldwide obesity epidemic, but heart disease and many other illnesses. But now, after years in the making, it's finally being recognized that not only are couch potatoes getting unhealthy; athletes also are.

The growing awareness includes athletes on all levels, including Olympians. Two conditions dominate: debilitating diseases referred to as chronic (meaning they've been simmering in an unhealthy body for years), and also, the real but sensitive issue of too much body fat.

There's a giant McDonald's in the heart of London's Olympic Park—in fact, it's the world's largest McDonald's and can seat fifteen hundred hungry people. The golden arches and Olympic gold seem to go hand in hand, and hardly anyone notices. Once the Games are over, the McDonald's will be torn down, but not before serving three million people.

And what is the message being sent to athletes as well? That you can be fit but also unhealthy?

In the 2007 U.S. marathon trials, Ryan Shay, one of America's best and a favorite for the Olympic team, collapsed and died about five miles into the race. It was sad, of course, any way we look at it. Ryan had a heart attack. But why were so many people confused about the death of such a great athlete at age twenty-eight? New York City's Chief Medical Examiner, who added to the confusion with his report, said the cause of Shay's death was, "cardiac arrhythmia due to cardiac hypertrophy with patchy fibrosis of undetermined etiology. Natural causes." Natural causes? There's nothing natural about a young, very fit athlete whose heart stops during competition.

Today, news reports of athletes dying in the course of competition are too common. Tragically, not long afterward, a forty-three-year-old male competitor died in the first ever New York City Ironman triathlon after suffering a heart attack during the 2.4-mile swim section in the Hudson River. While we take physical injury and health risks as an intrinsic element of participatory sports, we're bewildered when a seemingly healthy Ironman athlete drops dead. But healthy people don't have heart attacks.

Alberto Salazar, currently a distance coach for Nike and former national and world champion from 5K to the marathon, was moments away from death when his heart attack hit at forty-eight years young. Salazar asked his cardiologist, Todd Caulfield, MD, Provident St. Vincent Medical Center in Portland, Oregon, to speak publicly about his condition, which included previous medications for high blood pressure and cholesterol, which could not prevent the heart attack.

Hank Gathers, Jim Fixx, and many other very fit athletes from amateurs to professionals in all sports, and too many more whose names are not popular, have died or came close to death during training and competition.

Consider these two key factors:

- In most of these cases, athletes died of *preventable* conditions.
- In virtually all cases, there is an underlying unhealthy pathology.

In active individuals, prevention of heart disease, which is commonly accompanied by high blood fats and hypertension, can be primarily accomplished by a healthy diet. The Centers for Disease Control and Preventions (CDC) list four habits that cause preventable conditions such as heart disease: smoking, inactivity, alcohol abuse, and diet.

While most athletes don't have problems with the first three, they do have very poor eating habits.

But a serious problem is brewing. Is the world accepting of fit athletes dying at young ages? After all, in non-contact sports such as running, cycling, triathlon, and others, injuries are now considered part of the game, almost normal (which they are not). Overtraining may be the most common cause of chronic injuries, and not just physical impairments but those of a chemical nature (such as fatigue) and mental ones (depression).

As great as many athletes may be, reductions in their health will also impair their performance to some degree. How much better could even the best be if they were also healthy?

As American sprinter Manteo Mitchell got midway through the start of the four-hundred-meter relay, he felt, and heard, his leg crack. But he could not stop. Because it was not a weight-bearing bone, sprinting the best he could to finish his part of the relay enabled the American team to finish second and move on the finals (where they would get a silver medal without Mitchell).

A victory, no doubt, and an incredibly courageous effort by a young Olympian. Gutsy, heroic—and the made for TV moments for which the Olympic Games are often remembered. Afterwards Mitchell would find out the bone on the outside of his leg (the fibula) had fractured.

Without discounting Mitchell's valor, I can't help but think of something even more unsettling—why would a young, super-fit athlete's bone fracture during a short running event? Mitchell thought that perhaps his misstep while walking the stairs a few days earlier caused it. But leading up to the race, including his warm up, he ran without any problem.

Bones don't just break, especially in a young athlete, without some physiological reason. It could come from muscle or hormone imbalance or a combination of causes—some health problem contributed to a weak bone in a fit body.

Overfat Athletes

Looking at the broader picture, a much more sensitive and equally serious issue is that the "fat fallout" from the worldwide obesity epidemic has reached the athletic community. Perhaps for the first time, this Olympics has spawned a few controversial articles about overweight competitors, bringing to light the reality that fit but overfat athletes also exist.

Certainly those of us, like myself, who have worked with athletes for many years have seen this problem brewing for decades. The question will be whether the weekend warrior and recreational athletes will accept this overfat state.

While some athletes clearly have too much body fat—you can see it, and it's also been measured—others who appear slim have their fat elsewhere. Salazar is not an unusual case—some of his arteries were 80 percent clogged with fat.

Deep-pocketed gargantuan corporations selling junk food are not only making the entire world fat—they're exploiting athletes to help their propaganda succeed. Case in point: Coke celebrated the 2012 Olympics with specially marked cans, complete with eight teaspoons of sugar for each twelve-ounce serving. A key message of soft drink and other junk food companies is that sugar—one of the main causes of the overfat epidemic—is good for everyone.

The very companies that sponsor the Olympics—and the many high-profile sports events regularly broadcast throughout the world on a regular basis—are doing a lot of the dirty work. McDonald's and Coca-Cola are banking on the fact that their Olympic marketing campaigns will be highly successful—particularly with children and teens who, these companies hope, will become life-long customers.

The same marketing tactics were used by cigarette brand Virginia Slims. The cigarette company sponsored athletic events—not just tennis but even a New York City 10K running race—for years before lawsuits prevented tobacco companies from advertising in print, TV, and radio. Is there anyone (apart from Big Tobacco) who can't see the conflict of interest here?

The conflict of interest is just as obvious in companies that advertise sugar-laden soft drinks and other junk food during the Olympics. But the level of acceptance with these unhealthy food products is not yet like that of tobacco.

Society cannot keep avoiding the obvious and continue allowing companies to reap financial benefits by selling harmful products—the very foods that significantly contribute to heart disease and other deadly conditions—while portraying slim, healthy-looking individuals using the products. In the 1950s, doctors were seen in magazine print ads claiming that smoking cigarettes was actually good for you.

But the cries about junk food are only starting to be heard. While society has accepted Coke and McDonald's, and the hundreds of other companies making deadly products, there may be hope. A movement has been underway by people who want to ban the sale of unhealthy products in places like schools, cities, and even countries. At the same time, these efforts are heavily countered by the junk food industry's millions of lobbying dollars.

In the meantime, prime time TV will continue portraying athletes who are fit, and not necessarily healthy. And sadly, more stories of athletes' deaths from preventable conditions will be reported, too.

Asthma: the most common chronic medical condition of Olympians

Another example of fit but unhealthy athletes is asthma, a chronic respiratory condition characterized by episodes or attacks of impaired breathing. Symptoms are caused by chronic inflammation and narrowing of the airways going into and out of the lungs. Shortness of breath, coughing, wheezing, and chest pain are the most common complaints of asthmatics.

Asthma is a treatable condition—I'm not talking about using drugs to treat symptoms, but improving the overall health of the body to eliminate the problem. (Of course, proper medication may sometimes be temporarily needed for some patients, but with improving health, the reduction, and then elimination, of drug therapy can occur when it's no longer necessary.)

Many environmental triggers are known to activate asthmatic symptoms, such as cold air, chlorine, food, and other allergies—and even working out (leading to the so-called "exercise-induced asthma"), but these don't *cause* asthma. Since it's difficult to say what really causes the condition (we know it's not genetics), we have to take a different approach in helping patients with the problem—that is to improve overall health.

In general, healthy people don't have asthma. So improving the overall health of those who do have the condition can help eliminate it. That's been my approach in treating many patients with asthma. The two most common remedies include:

- Eliminating refined carbohydrates.
- Taking the nutrient choline (discussed below).

Of course, it could be said that most health conditions—from the majority of physical injuries and intestinal problems to fatigue and high blood pressure—could be successfully eliminated when the individual significantly improves his or her overall health.

The Centers for Disease Control and Prevention (CDC) report that about 8 percent of American adults have asthma. But in some sports, especially the endurance community, there is a much higher incidence of the condition.

Recent data collected by Pascale Kippelen and colleagues at Brunel University, Uxbridge, UK, and a number of other universities worldwide (*British Journal of Sports Medicine*, 2012), showed that in the past five summer and winter Olympic Games, about 8 percent of athletes had asthma (about the same as the general population). The study also showed the incidence of asthma in these particular sports:

- Cross country skiers 15 percent
- Swimmers and cyclists 17 percent

- Downhill skiers and divers 4 percent
- Triathletes 25 percent

Most of these Olympians used inhalers (beta 2-agonists), which dilate the bronchial passageways into the lungs to improve their breathing. Athletes taking asthma medications have consistently outperformed their peers (those who were not asthmatic and taking medication).

In 2009, the World Anti-Doping Agency (WADA) started removing asthma medications from its list of unapproved drugs. First was salbutamol; then, in 2012, formoterol was taken off this list. The reason is that, despite asthmatics on medication outperforming their peers, the WADA found the laboratory research linking these prescription drugs to improved performance was not sufficiently significant.

While research has not provided useful clues about the cause of asthma (probably because it's so variable and individual), many clinicians have. Throughout my career, asthma was not an uncommon complaint from athletes visiting my clinic. In most cases, eliminating the condition could be accomplished in those making the appropriate changes necessary to improve their health. These included dietary, environmental, stress, and other lifestyle factors.

Perhaps the three most common problems associated with asthma in these athletes included—overtraining, chronic inflammation, and carbohydrate intolerance. Although, in a clinical sense, as these three problems are usually interconnected, addressing only one or two health issues often did not reduce asthma symptoms. These topics are addressed in this book and in more detail in the two aforementioned Big books.

The Need for Choline

Choline is an essential nutrient, often associated with the B vitamins (but not officially defined as such). Aside from getting it from liver, the best food source is egg yolks. Choline supplementation is commonly required in higher amount in those individuals with asthma. Important for brain, muscle, and liver function, choline can also help the nervous system control proper bronchial action, perhaps due to its anti-inflammatory effects.

In most asthmatics I've treated, a moderate to high dose of supplemental choline may be needed initially—for example, 500 mg several times daily until breathing improves and dietary choline is increased.

Improving one's overall health is the best treatment for asthma. Although this is an individual issue, overtraining, chronic inflammation, and carbohydrate intolerance may be the three most common problems in athletes with asthma.

The Ultimate Athlete: Paleo People Today

Who are the world's ultimate athletes? Are they the East Africans infringing on a 1:59 marathon? The best Ironman champions?

No doubt we can all name various sports and individuals who achieve amazing feats in them. But the answer is that we are all the ultimate athletes in the human race. Some are better balanced, more fit, run faster, or jump higher. The healthiest ones with great endurance may survive best.

No doubt many people are familiar with today's paleo patterns of living. These include being barefoot, eating healthy animal protein and fat, and avoiding modern manufactured junk food. Thanks to books such as *The Paleo Solution* by Robb Wolf, and the research of Dr. Loren Cordain and the outpouring of information by many others, millions of people are reaping the benefits of Paleolithic life as we know it.

Neither was it always an easy topic to discuss, nor is it novel—although the popular term "paleo" is relatively new. The awareness that humans have deviated from our ancestral habits goes back to Hippocrates, or earlier in China, and more recently books started emphasizing these ideas in the 1800s. In 1958, the bestselling book *Eat Fat to Get Slim* became popular. For me, it was well known among nutrition-oriented folk in the 1960s that refined carbohydrates, including sugar, were deadly.

Many lifestyle habits of human ancestors were quite similar for several million years, but deviating from them today can affect our genes, body, and mind in many unhealthy ways. A relatively recent change in diet beginning about five to ten thousand years ago demonstrated this break with the past, as the shift to more refined carbohydrates and inactivity led to chronic disease and today's worldwide overfat epidemic.

Unfortunately, today's paleo impact on the population is relatively small, with most not really living it—more see it as a "diet" rather than a way of life. It's overshadowed by the much larger overfat epidemic, which is still growing and affecting the masses around the globe. Even in areas of the world where starvation was the mainstay just one generation ago, the nutrition transition has suddenly made obesity the much larger problem.

While there's no doubt about the benefits of being barefoot for better body mechanics, avoiding all high glycemic food to reduce body fat and disease, and the wonders of natural paleo-type strength workouts, there's a serious component of the modern movement that's missing. It's an important feature of humanity that began in prehistoric times and helped get us to where we are today, and is a key evolutionary factor humans had before language—music.

Darwin on Music

Frogs do it, so do whales, and even mice—everyone knows birds do it. It's music. Human songs are a powerful neuro-stimulant that led to the development of language, helped match the best mates, and played a role in building better brains.

When we listen to music, our whole brain "lights up," unlike it does with virtually any other sensation. This, many believe, enabled early human brains to continually evolve into the most magnificent of biological structures.

Music was, and still is, an essential part of the human ability to communicate. For our ancestors, communicating with fellow paleos to keep the group safe let that cute man or woman on the rock know you're there, or just to stake out a territory was a survival skill closely connected with music. It's not really any different today, although our situation is different—society has changed, and many have lost music.

Music is referenced often in anthropological literature:

- Music appeared in the earliest humans some six million years ago, and played a vital role in Paleolithic people's survival and evolution. Archeologist Steven Mithen (*The Singing Neanderthals: The Origins of Music, Language, Mind and Body*." London: Weidenfeld & Nicolson) wrote that the increasingly complex lives of human ancestors required an increasingly complex yet "holistic'" vocal communication system, which he identifies as music.
- As Aniruddh Patel states in the article "Music, biological evolution, and the brain" (The Neurosciences Institute, San Diego, CA 2010), "one can predict with some confidence that the few remaining uncontacted tribes of humans, when finally described by anthropologists, will have music as part of their behavioral repertoire." I would add that, because of music's intuitive mathematical foundation, that it's universal—the same might be true of our first encounter with extraterrestrial life— music will be a common feature that helps us communicate. That musical knowledge is not learned but innate is a popular notion. Babies relate to it well. And, how else could the Beatles have created such great music without any musical knowledge of notes, time signatures or other basic theory?
- Music is clearly associated with emotions too. In early humans, the emotional centers of the brain may have evolved from the stimulation of songs. In addition to individuals, group emotions developed as a few or more sang to protect their territories, and prepared to defend it if necessary. We can further speculate that individual emotion was very much related to sexual

selection. E. G. Burrows wrote, "Where an emotion may be either individual or collective, it is the collective aspect that finds expression in song." (*Songs of Uvea and Futuna. Honolulu: Bernice P. Bishop Museum Bulletin* No. 183, 1945).

- Archeologists Edward Hagen and Peter Hammerstein ("Did Neanderthals and other early humans sing?") wrote, "A vocal signal can advertise both location and 'quality' to members of the opposite sex."

Among the early scientific observations on the evolution of music were those of Charles Darwin. Two key principles in his theory of evolution included the popular notion of natural selection and, separately, sexual selection, which is related to music.

Favorable survival characteristics—such as improved running ability or strength—of an individual are preserved in the offspring, as those possessing these features will most likely live longer and reproduce more. In *Origins of Species*, Darwin wrote, "This preservation of favorable individual differences and variations, and the destruction of those which are injurious, I have called Natural Selection, or the Survival of the Fittest."

Music was of vital importance in the relationship between male and female, and the process of choosing the best mate. Darwin referred to this as sexual selection.

Regarding music's role in human evolution, Darwin noted that "as neither the enjoyment nor the capacity of producing musical notes are faculties of the least direct use to man in reference to his ordinary habits of life, they must be ranked among the most mysterious with which he is endowed."

While the idea of a shared origin for language and music is pre-Darwinian, dating at least as far back as French enlightenment writings in the 1700s, the first evolutionary theory for music was presented by Darwin in *The Descent of Man* in 1871. Darwin drew an analogy with birdsong and theorized that music arose in our ancestors via mechanisms of sexual selection. He wrote: "Musical tones and rhythm were used by the half-human progenitors of man, during the season of courtship, when animals of all kinds are excited by the strongest passions." Darwin speculated that word-less courtship songs predated our linguistic abilities, and that such singing provided the foundation for the development of language.

Of course, without the proper nutrition, and the ability to obtain it with successful hunting, the singing stimulus would not, by itself, allow the brain to develop into such a great structure.

In many ways, early Paleolithic life revolved around these three aspects: hunting, gathering, and music. They were key parts of regular daily life.

Hence, a more important need arose for protein and fat from meat—both vital for optimal brain development—during the early Paleolithic period. The modern human brain, in addition to its high reliance on protein, is more than 60 percent fat.

While the combination of mating and territorial relationships to human song is more obvious, the drawing of people together could have helped larger groups of individuals and families in a single, defined territory begin a social structure. This further encouraged group hunting, where music was an integral part because it resulted in more success. The additional availability of meat as a quality food source further fed the brain's development to a more complex structure, continuing the process that led to Paleolithic people today.

Got Rhythm?

Paleolitic people developed something unique from other animals—a highly specialized, complex area of the brain called the cerebellum. This is the part that generates rhythm in the physical body. As a key component of more complex songs, rhythm in early humans not only made music more specialized, and those possessing it perhaps more attractive, but it also would have further assisted in successful mating, and improved hunting to help provide more nutrition for those little paleos.

As the brain developed a greater degree of complexity and synchronization of rhythm, the better the quality of the coalition in protecting territory and mates (and children) would have lead to even more group strength.

The brain's rhythm directly affects muscles. A cerebellum would have led to better, more effective physical activity. Dance evolved from rhythm, too, becoming an important social feature of early humans, and another way to form alliances with other groups or tribes. Humans would literally choose their friends and allies wisely based on musical quality.

So for early humans, music appeared to help attract allies, indicate territory ownership, attract the best mates, improve hunting success, and discourage enemies. Is there any question it would be good for paleo people today?

As the human brain, body, and civilization itself continued evolving, music became more than a method for matching mates and protecting territory. It became an important cultural component, with entertainment evolving too. This human trait maintains its high level of importance in sexuality today.

For millions of years, music was both brain and body oriented. Triggering excitement of the hunt—an animal to eat or a mate that matched—music was as important as the paleo diet. Humans were thoroughly engaged by their music, not simply mildly entertained—herein lies one of the problems with today's paleo people.

Today we are in the age of communication breakdown, despite all the high-tech devices. It all began just recently, it seems, with the popularity of the telephone in the mid-twentieth century. With the phone, we no longer needed to talk face-to-face. This evolved into faxes, pagers and, of course, emails, texting, and tweets.

For humans, face-to-face contact is a foundation of communication. It's so important that our brain evolved to devote large amounts of space and energy to vision (a reason musicians often close their eyes during performance—it reduces activity of the brain's visual areas devoting more energy to performing). In particular, communicating long-distances with songs, say scientists, led to more modern music. We can hear similar statements from today's animals too. Consider the howling of wolves and screeches of hawks from a distance during hunting and courting.

Along with communication and sexual selection, humans also made music to mark their territories. While some animals, like cats, mark their territory with scents, early humans did not and instead used sounds. Music was the human form of scent.

Humans would eventually evolve to sing duets. This is a most unique animal feature (although a few modern-day birds do this), which gradually became more complex and coordinated, and sung by male and female. In addition to advertising each partner's newfound physical territory, singing together further signaled the couple's status to rivals, an announcement of the committed relationship.

In addition to singing with their mates, early humans may have defended their territory in groups, with compelling, coordinated vocalizations to mark their ownership. Perhaps this was the first rock band.

All humans were rock stars—actually, it was more folk music, from which most musical genres today were derived. Everyone in the clan was musical, unlike today where a significant separation of musical and non-musical people began to appear just a few hundred years ago.

Long before musical instruments, songs were sung by all individuals, eventually with vocal choruses by others, and then leading to harmony and other sounds as specialized brain areas developed. Combined with the expanding brain, human anatomy would have also allowed different oral resonances, various singing sounds such as humming, whistling, blowing, and groaning (not unlike what many vocalists do today). This would have evolved to percussive sounds as the brain's cerebellum developed to provide better tempo—perhaps just banging bones or stones, clapping hands, or slapping skin—and no doubt beating their chests.

As the brain evolved and complex vocalizations developed, the more detailed recognizable pitch of individual notes was emphasized over humming, whistling, and groaning. This would be an important foundation for the development of language.

The invention of non-percussion instruments would not come until, presumably, millions of years later. Archeologists recently found the oldest human instrument to date in a German cave—a 42,000-year-old bird bone flute. This was the period humans were migrating out of Africa into Europe, and music was more highly developed and powerful. Perhaps this was the first pied piper? A human making music from a bone must have had a large fan-base following him or her.

The mass migration to all parts of the earth spawned many different cultures—none of which were without music. And every human culture had some form of music with a periodic beat pattern, to which people synchronize their rhythmic movements whether for procreation, hunting, fighting, dancing, or running.

Today, music has become solely a body experience for many, one of thumping drum beats that rev you up to get through that morning workout. It's something many attempt to use to keep out the noise and other stresses of modern life—or to break the sound of silence in the elevator. But for millions of years, and through the 1960s, music was much more. It was a cultural expression, and, most importantly, a powerful experience for the evolving brain—it's what being human was all about.

As paleo people today, it's important for us to consider not only one's diet, but also all other features that fed the brains of our ancestors. Along with hunting and gathering, the music of the earliest humans played an integral part in helping them survive and evolve.

Surviving Athletic Extinction

Each year, scientists warn us, tens of thousands of species become extinct. As most agree, it is just a matter of time for humans to fall prey to such a natural cycle. While human technology may have created an irreversible mess of our planet—not only the environment, but also the people who are part of it—we must find a way to use high tech to save us. Of course, no one has all the answers about how this might be done. However, the real issue is whether enough healthy humans can survive what many say is the process of extinction that has already begun.

Our planet's past includes many instances of mass devastations that wiped out large numbers of inhabitants. Scientists tell us there have been five major mass extinctions, where most of life disappeared. And except for one event, when earth was nearly destroyed in a short period after being struck by a large meteor, the rest took place over many thousands of years. During these extinctions, it was typical for about 75 percent of life on earth to disappear. While there have been many other less-discussed and smaller scale extinctions, the sixth major devastation, scientists say, has already started. Which of today's paleo people will survive? The answer is obvious: those who are more physically and mentally healthy will be most capable of carrying on humanity.

The current extinction may have started about fifty thousand years ago. Called the Pleistocene extinction, it first involved paleo people killing too many animals to meet their growing need for food. Today, we can raise enough animals, but pollution and poor health have become the primary causes of our apparent and rapidly accelerating demise. Of course, these problems are strictly preventable; but most humans choose to look the other way as the process of mass extinction continues.

Let's not even discuss the possibility of being hit by a large enough meteor to demolish the planet. How many people would survive just a loss of electrical power? Imagine not being able to use your kitchen or car, heat or air conditioning, or most other modern conveniences? But this problem pales in comparison to the existing crises already upon us. More significant is the global health disaster, in which 75 percent of the population is overfat. In addition to the gross burden of costs, and the possible plummeting of social structure, this condition significantly affects fertility. I've addressed these issues in past books and articles.

Now we are hearing another key clue. Suddenly, music itself may be warning us about our extinction.

When the Music's Over

Among the species undergoing rapid extinction today are songbirds. And scientists have discovered something that could also apply to humans.

The earliest humans produced music that dramatically improved their reproductive success, helped in the search for food, the development of society, and overall survival. Music may be the only single stimulation that turns on all the many areas of the brain, helping it to function optimally in so many ways, including creativity and maintaining a healthy body.

But when a species faces extinction, one warning sign may include diminishing song quality. Scientists have discovered this phenomenon in certain types of songbirds. Other researchers have shown a sudden and unique change in human music over the last twenty years, too—changes frighteningly similar to those of the disappearing songbirds.

In addition to changes in song quality, more humans than ever have lost their musicality. Many not only don't play or sing, something unheard of just a few hundred years ago, but some are also even averse to music's natural stimulation. Delegated to the background, but popular in elevators and driving forces of games, music's role as a commercial vehicle is most popular in selling us all those unnecessary things that pollute the air and airways.

Today, unwanted sound—noise—is interfering with nature. We know this is another problem for songbirds, but humans are also drowning in a sea of noise. This has an adverse effect on the brain, and poses a serious stress that further impairs our health.

Noise pollution—from auto, train, bus and air traffic, to machinery, radio, TV, and Internet chatter—can seriously impair our ability to benefit from songs we might hear.

In their attempt to adapt to unnatural noisy environments, songbirds change the frequencies of their songs, one of the factors associated with reduced quality, which can reduce the effectiveness in triggering female responses. Too much noise in the environment can cause a decline in the number of breeding bird territories, and reduced reproductive success.

What Can Paleo People Do?

Is the earth's extreme pollution problem beyond repair? Are more people functioning in inhumane ways? Whether the answers to these questions are obvious or not, it still comes down to one key issue: we are responsible for our own health and fitness—and survival. All humans have this instinct built-in to the genes. Saving the planet, and humanity, starts with each of us as individuals.

Along with some luck, the 25 percent of the population that may survive mass extinctions does so because they are the healthiest and most fit. It's also possible these are the most musical people, too. Just as in Paleolithic times, our songs remain as important as proper nutrition and optimal endurance.

When it comes to making music part of a healthy life, there's nothing complicated about it. When stopping to smell the roses, we hear the music, too.

Hearing, seeing, and playing music is therapeutic for the brain and body. Just take the time to listen. Do it in your car, sit with a few songs while having morning coffee, with your meals and in other situations—make it a part of your life again. Instead of watching the news or other TV, listen to an album each evening while relaxing. Find the music that makes you feel good. For many people, these are the songs from yesterday—from a time when life seemed more simple, relaxing and fun. This might be the music of your teen years, or the songs you first fell in love with. But the brain loves new music too, and there's plenty of it out there when you weed through the junk. (In addition, get that old guitar out of the closet or dust off the piano—and just play!)

Putting all the scientific stuff aside, the simplest way to know how the paleo process applies to you is you: how do you feel from the lifestyle you live each day considering diet and activity? And, does the music you hear move you? It should. It is not a separate musical feature for the brain, as songs are shown to improve all the non-musical areas, too (probably through changes in consciousness, that is to say the production of alpha waves, blood circulation, and hormone regulation).

Paleolithic people were holistic, and, today we are meant to be the same, particularly if we want to live life to the fullest and survive as a species.

The Modern Myth of Holistic Health

It's cool to use the word *holistic*. And it's exploited in most areas of health-related products and services, from dietary supplements and cosmetics to therapies of all types. Many people consider themselves to be holistic when it comes to healthcare because they do something associated with the term. This might be getting an acupuncture treatment, a chiropractic adjustment, taking herbs, or even shopping at a health-food store. But this is certainly not what holistic is all about.

The term holistic is not synonymous with so-called alternative therapies, nor organic food or fair trade, although that's often how it's used. And, it's not necessarily part of the mind-body movement that's been popularized in recent years. The way most of these activities are utilized—actually quite narrow in scope—is far from what holistic is all about.

Music therapy is not holistic. Neither is kinesiology, cranial osteopathy, or American Indian dance, although most people involved in these and similar routines consider their participation in them as a holistic act.

The term holistic is not well defined. Much like the word *natural*, it's often used to impress others, lure consumers, or to help people feel comfort, especially when selling a service.

Here's how I define holistic: It's the understanding that everything in life effects us—the food we eat, our physical activity, society, and all aspects of our environment. And it's the knowledge that we have control of these factors to the extent that, by managing it well we can significantly influence our health. In other words, with very few exceptions, we are in charge of our health.

The foundation of being holistic is living it—eating and being physically active is only part of it. Thinking it in a way that promotes optimal brain and bodily function is just as important. It's striving to be in balance in all we do all the time. Humans have evolved along with the environment, so we also must maintain a healthy world—all of our surroundings in the living environment, including the air we breathe, what we sense, see, feel, smell, and hear.

All this affects our brains, how we think and feel, and behavior—so holism includes our mental and emotional health too, and beyond to include the individual's spiritual beliefs, however difficult to understand.

Separate from this are the many therapeutic tools that can positively influence our health, although none can make up for a poor diet, inactivity or an unbalanced environment. They might include various treatments from acupuncture and manipulation to nutrition and biofeedback, including those associated with improving brain function. These activities are only adjuncts to the foundation of living a holistic life. The more solid this foundation, the less we require outside intervention because, overall, a healthy body and brain can keep us more balanced than any therapy.

All this is a difficult pill to swallow in a society that's obsessed about focusing on one small part of an issue or trend while brushing aside and ignoring the rest of the important factors. As an example, many people go on a diet while remaining physically inactive. Others regularly visit various types of health care practitioners to treat end-result symptoms instead of improving their overall health and environment.

Doctors, nurses, and other healthcare practitioners can significantly influence how people think about the concept of holism. Based on surveys, those practitioners who were considered holistic had more spiritual and/or religious beliefs, and utilized some form of alternative techniques compared to general practitioners. More mainstream medical practitioners are now believing the word holistic should be spelled 'wholistic' to avoid confusion with complementary and alternative medicine.

Of course, these words are also thrown around like an old pair of running shoes: the term 'alternative' has a more radical definition, inferring an exclusive use of therapies that are not mainstream medicine. Many believe that one is either alternative in his or her healthcare approach, or follow the modern medical model of treating symptoms (but in reality, most people yield to both). But the fact is, most alternative therapies today follow the same symptom-based model.

The term "complementary" refers to a more open or holistic view that we have the option of using any and all approaches that might help us—from nutrition or biofeedback, to drugs or surgery. Relying on more conservative approaches as much as possible, knowing other options exist, is typically holistic.

Not only does our healthcare education encourage practitioners to not be holistic, the standards of care in virtually all professions make it illegal. Going into private practice in 1977 in New York State meant I could not be holistic unless I broke the law. Not knowing any other way to effectively care for individuals, I went beyond my legal scope of practice almost daily. It was key to helping people in their quest to be healthy and fit. And no one ever complained.

Throughout the world today, there are few truly holistic-healthcare models. A model is a format, or an approach to patient care, and just the opposite of a cookbook routine. The most effective models are those that rely on assessment to find, and address, the cause of health problems.

The modern healthcare system further breaks down because patients generally choose their own therapies based on symptoms. For example, if you have low back pain, you may go to a chiropractor. But what if the cause of your pain is not solely a spinal misalignment? What if the problem is also associated with inflammation of the spinal joints? In this case, two therapies might be necessary to resolve the back pain—spinal manipulation and dietary and nutritional recommendations to help control inflammation. Or, if three or four techniques are necessary to resolve the cause of the problem, this further complicates things, unless one particular practitioner has expertise in assessing and applying the proper therapies, which is possible.

Healthcare practitioners who encourage patients to participate in the process of improving and maintaining their health may be part of an ideal holistic relationship. The word *doctor* means *teacher*—this education is a powerful tool, enabling many individuals to learn more about their bodies, and obtain high levels of wellness just by taking care of themselves through optimal diet, physical activity, balancing their environment, and other habits that form the foundation of health.

Today's healthcare system shuns the holistic approach, one of the reasons it has failed. It is really disease care, and does not encourage people to take responsibility for their health but await symptoms to arise and treat them. But individuals who are holistic are changing the system by addressing the causes of preventable diseases—from Alzheimer's and cancer to heart disease and physical ailments—by eating well, being active, building better brain function, creating a balanced environment, and having a higher quality of life.

Dangers for Today's Paleo Athletes

By now you know the dangers encountered by modern human athletes. Food and inactivity are the two primary ones. There are many examples, but a recent item got my attention.

Junk Food Giant Nestlé Seeking "Exercise in a Bottle"

It's bad enough that junk food companies have contributed to a worldwide overfat epidemic, which has not spared athletes. They also helped mesmerize millions to become couch potatoes. Now the world's largest food company is spending $1.5 billion to find a formula they can bottle that contains a chemical to stimulate the body's metabolism like that of a workout.

In the November 24, 2014, edition of the journal *Chemistry & Biology*, scientists from the Nestlé Institute of Health Sciences in Lausanne, Switzerland, found that an enzyme that regulates the body's metabolism to burn sugars and fats can be controlled by a chemical called C13. The company is betting that the lucky compound can become a food additive, a magic bullet that could mimic the benefits of exercise. The no pain, no strain beverage will certainly contain lots of sugar.

Nestlé's scientists are searching for natural substances that could trigger C13 in the body. And they are looking for them in none other than natural plant foods. Those of us who consume natural plant foods as a significant part of a healthy diet are already reaping these benefits.

While $1.5 billion seems like a lot to throw at long-term risky research, Nestlé's annual revenue is around $100 billion. Their stock profile states that they are a nutrition, health, and wellness company, which manufactures, supplies, and produces prepared dishes, milk-based products, pharmaceuticals, baby foods, and cereals. With brands from Gerber and Kit Kat to Boost and Häagen-Dazs, many households are full of their processed foods.

Many other food companies have jumped on the so-called natural products bandwagon. Especially amid the recent surge in sales of healthy junk food items not only in many retail outlets, but even in restaurants.

In a trend to help create the perception of junk food being healthier, protein has become one of the hottest items. But since protein costs are high, manufacturers are countering this by using highly processed, cheap protein from soy, rice, and milk (typically in isolated, caseinated, and hydrolyzed forms, which may also contain monosodium glutamate, MSG). In grocery stores, 20 percent of new product introductions in 2012 were protein-related, including such junk food cereal items such as *Cheerios Protein*. Even restaurants are jumping in, with menus that claim rises in protein of 67 percent in the last five years.

Claims of cardio in a can may seem futuristic, but Nestlé says the new product could benefit diabetics, obese people, and others who are too unhealthy, unable, and unwilling to work out. But these are the very conditions the junk food industry created to begin with—and there may be billions of such people.

Balancing health and fitness is something we should all be striving to do. It takes logic, common sense, critical thinking, and most importantly, avoiding the hype of the latest craze. Run, ride, ski, walk, and swim intelligently. You can even do them all, if you listen to your body. And most importantly, have fun.

A REVIEW OF THE 180 FORMULA

To find your maximum aerobic training heart rate, there are two important steps. First, subtract your age from 180. Next, find the best category for your present state of fitness and health, and make the appropriate adjustments:

1. Subtract your age from 180.
2. Modify this number by selecting among the following categories the one that best matches your fitness and health profile:
   a. If you have or are recovering from a major illness (heart disease, any operation or hospital stay, etc.) or are on any regular medication, subtract an additional ten.
   b. If you are injured, have regressed in training or competition, get more than two colds or bouts of flu per year, have allergies or asthma, or if you have been inconsistent or are just getting back into training, subtract an additional five.
   c. If you have been training consistently (at least four times weekly) for up to two years without any of the problems just mentioned, keep the number (180 minus age) the same.

d. If you have been training for more than two years without any of the problems listed above, and have made progress in competition without injury, add five.

For example, if you are thirty years old and fit into category (b), you get the following:

180–30=150. Then 150–5=145 beats per minute (bpm).

In this example, 145 will be the highest heart rate for all training. This is highly aerobic, allowing you to most efficiently build an aerobic base. Training above this heart rate rapidly incorporates anaerobic function, exemplified by a shift to burning more sugar and less fat for fuel.

If it is difficult to decide which of two groups best fits you, choose the group or outcome that results in the lower heart rate. In athletes who are taking medication that may affect their heart rate, those who wear a pacemaker, or those who have special circumstances not discussed here, further individualization with the help of a health-care practitioner or other specialist familiar with your circumstance and knowledgeable in endurance sports may be necessary.

Two situations may be exceptions to the above calculations:

- The 180 Formula may need to be further individualized for people over the age of sixty-five. For some of these athletes, up to ten beats may have to be added for those in category (d) in the 180 Formula, and depending on individual levels of fitness and health. This does not mean ten should automatically be added, but that an honest self-assessment is important.
- For athletes sixteen years of age and under, the formula is not applicable; rather, a heart rate of 165 may be best.

Once a maximum aerobic heart rate is found, a training range from this heart rate to ten beats below could be used as a training range. For example, if an athlete's maximum aerobic heart rate is determined to be 155, that person's aerobic training zone would be 145 to 155 bpm. However, the more training at 155, the quicker an optimal aerobic base will be developed.

THE MAXIMUM AEROBIC FUNCTION (MAF) TEST

In addition to monitoring your workouts to assure you stay aerobic, another advantage of using a heart-rate monitor is the ability to objectively measure these improvements using the maximum aerobic function test, or MAF Test. I developed this evaluation in the early 1980s so athletes could more precisely monitor their progress—and, even more important, be alerted if their training was faltering or leading to an injury or overtraining.

The MAF Test can be performed with any endurance activity. Your goal is to measure how fast you can run, bike, swim, inline skate, and so on, over a given distance at your aerobic maximum heart rate. Alternatively, you can measure how far you can go in a given time frame at the same heart rate. You need not perform the MAF Test in your particular sport. A basketball or tennis player will observe that he or she can excel during play without the heart rate rising as much, but this is difficult to measure. Using other training methods, such as a stationary bike or treadmill, makes for a better MAF Test.

During the MAF Test, use your maximum aerobic heart rate as determined by the 180 Formula. Using this heart rate, determine some parameter such as pace (minutes per mile), speed (miles per hour), or repetitions (laps in a pool) over time. The test can also be done on stationary equipment measuring watts, for example, if the equipment is accurate.

To perform a MAF Test during running, for example, the use of a quarter mile or a four hundred-meter running track is ideal. A three-to-five mile distance provides more information. All MAF Tests should be done following a warm-up (discussed later). The following is an actual MAF Test performed by a runner on a track, calculating time in minutes per mile:

Mile 1   8:21
Mile 2   8:27
Mile 3   8:38
Mile 4   8:44
Mile 5   8:49

As indicated by the above chart, it's normal to obtain slightly slower times with each ensuing mile (which demonstrates a normal fatigue factor). The slower your first mile, the more the time will slow between the first and fifth mile. This is due to reduced aerobic function, which is associated with lower endurance. If your first mile is a 10:17 pace, for example, your fifth mile could be 11:20. On the other hand, if your first mile is faster, the difference between miles one and five is less—if your first mile is 5:50, your fifth mile may be 6:14.

During any one MAF Test, it's normal for your times to get slower; the first mile should always be the fastest, and the last the slowest. If that's not the case, it usually means your warm-up was inadequate. An example of this is if your first mile is 7:46 and your second is 7:39. In addition, as the weeks pass, the MAF Test should show faster times compared to previous tests. The chart below shows typical endurance progress in the same runner from chart above:

	April	May	June	July
Mile 1	8:21	8:11	7:57	7:44
Mile 2	8:27	8:18	8:05	7:52
Mile 3	8:38	8:26	8:10	7:59
Mile 4	8:44	8:33	8:17	8:09
Mile 5	8:49	8:39	8:24	8:15

I refer to these improvements as *aerobic speed*—the development of a faster running pace, cycling speed, or other endurance improvements that occur during the aerobic base training. During periods of anaerobic training, including the competitive season, improvements in speed at the same heart rate usually slow or stop. This means that aerobic development is slowing or stopping, which may be normal and temporary.

Most important, and one of the key factors regarding the MAF Test, is that if you don't make progress during this base building period or, if after some improvements, your MAF Test begins to worsen, it usually indicates there is a problem with your training, diet, stress management, or another factor impairing your aerobic system. This should serve as a significant warning. It may be associated with the onset of a cold or other illness, a dietary problem such as eating poorly during the holiday season, a nutritional problem such as anemia, excess stress from your job, or the early stage of overtraining. Often, an athlete determines an incorrect maximum aerobic training heart rate from the 180 Formula, making the heart rate too high. Even slight elevations—such as three beats—may eventually cause the aerobic system to not progress. This is a critical aspect of endurance training as the MAF Test is telling you something is wrong. Evaluating your physical, chemical, and mental stresses—from other physical work to diet and mental stress—is essential to not only get your fitness back on track to build endurance, but to prevent your health from faltering.

The MAF Test in Other Sports

The MAF Test is the most important self-administered assessment tool for endurance athletes. It's something to evaluate about once a month throughout the year. I described how runners can use the MAF Test above. Performing the Test on a bike is similar in concept to running, except cyclists have various ways to record results. The best and easiest method is to measure power at your maximum aerobic heart rate. another method is to pick a flat bike course that takes about thirty to forty-five minutes to complete. Following a warm-up, ride at your maximum aerobic heart rate, and record exactly how long it takes to ride the test course. As you progress with more speed, your times should get lower. Riding your course today, for example, may take 36:50. A month later it may take you 35:30 and after another month, 34:15. After three months of base work, the same course may only take you thirty-three minutes.

Still another option is to ride on a flat course and see how fast a pace you can maintain while holding your heart rate at your maximum aerobic level. This works best in a velodrome, or indoors on a training apparatus. As you progress, your speed should increase. If you start at eighteen mph, for example, following a three-month period of building aerobic base, you could be riding twenty-four mph at the same heart rate.

Cross-country skiers can follow a similar routine to evaluate their MAF tests.

For swimmers, the same idea for the MAF Test is applied. In this case, you can use a pool or open water to evaluate aerobic progress. Because swimming is such a low gravity stress activity, you will find that aerobic speed builds quickly and will require more physical ability to keep up with the pace. In other words, you will have to swim much faster to keep your heart rate at the max aerobic rate—in many swimmers with good technique and endurance it may not be possible to maintain the max aerobic heart rate for a forty-minute workout, for example. While this is a sign of good endurance progress, it makes performing the MAF Test difficult. Until this happens, it's best to maintain faster swimming only if you can maintain good technique.

When you're not able to swim fast enough, or maintain good technique in the water, you have two options regarding MAF Test evaluation:

- First, you can perform your test at a lower heart rate. If your max aerobic heart rate is 150 but you physically can't swim fast enough to reach that rate without your technique suffering, use a heart rate that's more comfortable, 130 for example, if that allows you to swim with good technique.
- A second consideration is to use another activity to monitor aerobic progress. If you also ride a bike or run, use one (or both) of these sports to perform your MAF Test. Progression on a bike, which improves conversion of fat to energy and other aerobic system aspects, will also allow you to swim at a faster pace.

WATER INTOXICATION AND HYPONATREMIA

Drinking fluids during training and racing will soon be reaching a boiling point of controversy and not for reasons you might suspect. Dehydration, and how to keep it under control, is nothing new. What's been bubbling up in the media for the past few years is *hyperhydration*—drinking too much and how it can lead to ill health and death. It's also been called *water intoxication*. While the problem is usually associated with long hot races such as an Ironman triathlon, it can occur at any time given the right circumstances. Twenty-eight-year-old Jennifer Strange died in 2007 after competing in a Sacramento, California, radio show contest to see how much water contestants could consume. The local coroner said her condition was consistent with water intoxication. The problem has become one of the more serious risks in certain sports, as over-hydrated marathoners, triathletes, and ultra-endurance athletes have died during races or right afterward.

So what's going on? Because, as I will point out here, there soon might be limitations on the amount of water and sports drinks offered on race courses, with recommendations that athletes consume much less than what's been encouraged for years. In fact, the recommenda-tions of reduced water and sports drink intake already is emphasized in places like New Zealand and South Africa, where water intoxica-tion is not nearly the problem compared to North America.

But there's more to the issue. Certainly, the sports drink and bottled water industry has pushed the recommendations that more fluid is better while sponsoring many races and individual athletes. An even broader view of the issue is that athletes themselves influ-ence their risk of ill health and even death on race day in the way they train and the lifestyle they live. There's even a relationship with muscle balance, gait, and physical injuries. And, water intoxication comes with another serious, life-threatening condition called hypo-natremia—low blood sodium. Looking at the problems of hydration and sodium regulation must be done holistically as many factors can be to blame.

However, it's important for each athlete to individualize his or her own needs, based on body size, the particular race environment, and level of fitness. Even more important is that, if you're not healthy, racing is something to avoid since your risk of injury, worsening of health, and even serious emergency conditions, which can lead to death, are real consequences. The combination of water intoxication and hyponatremia is one grave example.

Improving your overall health, not just your fitness levels, and following some simple guidelines, such as not drinking fluids to excess, can improve the body's ability to regulate water, and its key electrolyte partner, sodium. Otherwise, you could *gain* weight during a long race and risk serious water and sodium imbalance.

Instead, endurance athletes are often encouraged to drink more during long training and racing. Much of this information comes from the very companies selling fluid replacement drinks, and often the same sponsors of races. The result is that, for many athletes it's turned into an obsession—not just during races. Many athletes carry a water bottle on their bike for short rides, some during a run, and the majority cling to one at work or when driving. An ever-present water bottle has become like a pacifier for adult athletes.

Drink up! has been the recommendation for decades, not just in hot weather, where the loss of fluid is great, but during long events with cool or even cold temperatures.

Why so much confusion? Through the many years of telling athletes drinking more is better, the research has been showing we can really drink too much Gatorade and other fancy drinks, including water. The answer is that it's a question of balance.

Proper hydration is key to this issue of not too much, not too little water. This means your fluid intake during a race should be about the same as your fluid loss.

Too Little=Dehydration

Fluid replacement is important during long races and training. It helps maintain blood volume, proper heart rate, blood flow in the skin to dissipate excess heat, and to prevent body temperature from rising too high, among other functions. A properly hydrated athlete will also subjectively feel the event is easier (a lower perception of effort), and will prevent the heart rate from climbing too high (a reflection of increased stress that will result in the athlete slowing down).

At the 2007 Chicago Marathon, a shortage of water on a hot day suddenly became a problem for the back-of-the pack runners and long before the halfway point. Fearing health concerns from dehydration, race officials shut down the race for many runners.

It wasn't too long ago that marathon courses and other long endurance events did not allow water stops or restricted fluids. During the 1904 St. Louis Olympic marathon, only one water stop was available, about midway through the course, although trainers did provide their runners with water along the way. Tour de France officials used to limit each rider to about two liters of water. However, during races, riders raided roadside bars for refreshments and filled their bottles from fountains.

In 1969, a study by C. H. Wyndham and N. B. Strydom entitled "The Danger of an Inadequate Water Intake During Marathon Running" in the *South African Medical Journal* may have been one of the triggers for new water recommendations, influencing international rule changes that would allow fluid intake—water stops—during endurance races.

By this point, Gatorade, created in 1965 for football players, began expanding into new markets—not just the world of jogging, which was becoming popular, but as a beverage for everyday use. The marathon craze in the 1970s and '80s further fueled the interest in energy drinks. As more people were involved with marathons and triathlons, race fluids became more widely and readily available. For example, Bud Light was the Hawaii Ironman title sponsor in the early 1980s, but afterwards it was Gatorade. The notion of "more is better" when it comes to fluid replacement was highlighted during race sponsorships. Most endurance events had an alliance with companies that sell sports drinks. This business relationship continues today as a billion-dollar industry. The main message of these companies to athletes—drink more!

Dehydration can be a serious health problem, and can even increase the risk of death. It can cause fatigue, nausea, weakness, muscle cramps, disorientation, slurred speech, and confusion. In the 1980 Hawaii Ironman event, race officials were concerned about safety, and so they instituted a weigh-in procedure. Triathletes were required to stop three times during the 112-mile bike section and once during the 26.2-mile run for body-weight measurements. These would be checked against one's recorded pre-race weigh-in. If a racer's weight went down by at least 10 percent, course officials would seek a mandatory withdrawal from competition.

But just six years later, the first published medical cases of a more serious problem for endurance athletes would be published—those that *gained* weight and had a severe drop in sodium. Too much water combined with low sodium would be shown to have serious and deadly consequences. Using the same weigh-in requirements today during the Ironman and similar races could save lives as the severity of the problem is usually associated with weight gain due to the high fluid intake and the body's inability to regulate water and sodium. About 25 percent of Ironman finishers are found to have abnormally low blood sodium.

The problem of hyponatremia, usually combined with water intoxication, is now referred to as *exercise associated hyponaturemia*—EAH (usually defined by blood levels of sodium less than 135 mmol/liter). It shows up in athletes during or within twenty-four hours of their race or training. When EAH is more advanced, the problem can produce edema in lungs and the brain. This serious condition, called *exercise associated hyponatremia encephalopathy* or EAHE, despite being uncommon, is one reason why so much is being made of water intoxication. EAHE not only can produce alterations in mental status and respiratory distress, but seizures, coma and death.

Too Much=Water Intoxication

In 1985, Dr. Timothy Noakes and colleagues published a groundbreaking research paper in the journal *Science and Medicine in Sports and Exercise*, which described the occurrence of water intoxication, too much body water, and hyponatremia, low blood sodium, in four endurance athletes competing for over seven hours. When advised to drink less fluid, three of the athletes subsequently completed the same type event without problems. Since this study, other researchers have studied the issues of hyperhydration and hyponatremia in detail, along with its causes, and the misconception that more water is better. Its acceptance in the sports world—heavily allied with the sports drink and bottled water industry—has been slow.

Since 2011, things have not changed too much. The acceptance of water intoxication, while mentioned in magazines and other media, has not always resulted in changes in race day encouragement of more fluid intake, although more medical directors at races are making the warning to not drink to excess. But a recent four-mile race in Sausalito, California, is an example of the continued promotion to drink more: their per-race literature boasts "several refreshment stations along the way"—with a water company as one of the sponsors. But for a four-mile fun run?

Even after a number of studies through the mid 1990s clearly demonstrated that over-drinking could cause serious health problems—including death—the subject was nearly ignored by many in the sports medicine world. Noakes writes in the *British Journal of Sports Medicine* (2010) that, "Instead, in 1996, influential guidelines of the ACSM [American College of Sports Medicine] promoted the concept that athletes should drink 'as much as tolerable' during exercise. What followed was an epidemic of cases of EAH and its associated encephalopathy (EAHE)." The new ACSM guidelines almost a decade later were essentially maintained, as Noakes noted: "It is instructive to review the industrial connections of those who wrote the 2007 ACSM Position Stand. Of the six authors, four . . . have direct and longstanding involvement with Gatorade."

Between 1993 and 2008, Tamara Hew-Butler and colleagues (published in the *Journal of Clinical Endocrinology and Metabolism,* 2008) state that five marathoners, four of them female, died from EAH. (Studies show that women athletes may be much more vulnerable to EAH.)

EAH can produce symptoms of fatigue, mental disorientation, gait alterations, breathing difficulty—or no symptoms at all making it difficult to diagnose, and differentiate it from dehydration, without the help of a trained healthcare professional.

In a study compiling 2,135 endurance athletes who completed forty-two-kilometer marathons, 109-kilometer cycling events, and 226-kilometer Ironman triathlons (*Proceedings of the National Academy of Sciences,* 2005), Noakes found that about 60 percent were dehydrated while 11 percent were overhydrated. Overall, 6 percent had mild hyponatremia, and 1 percent had severe hyponatremia.

Athletes who gain weight during long races or training may be considered overhydrated. Those who lose more than about 3 percent body weight may be considered dehydrated. Today, EAH is considered one of the most common life-threatening complications of endurance exercise.

Now, we're about to come full circle with new water and fluid recommendations for all athletes competing in endurance events. That is, if these guidelines aren't shut down or lobbied against by the companies selling these products; they are often major sponsors of races and athletes. Regardless of whether it's the cause or a contributory factor, excessive amounts of water intake can produce EAH and EAHE. So by restricting water and educating athletes to not drink excessively, these types of deaths can be prevented.

When it comes to drinking fluids, the tradition of "more is better" is not easy to break.

In a 2004 study of Ironman triathletes published in the *British Journal of Sports Medicine*, Karen Sharwood and colleagues concluded that, "There is a large body of literature that suggests that dehydration impairs performance and increases the risk of heat illness in ultra-distance races. However, these conclusions have been based on laboratory studies using exercise interventions of relatively short duration and are thus limited in their application to performance in the field." Sharwood's study was performed during the 2000 and 2001 South African Ironman Triathlon, and showed that there was no increased risk of heat illness associated with high levels of dehydration, and that high levels of weight loss do not significantly influence performance.

In fact, in some endurance events the top finishers showed some of the greatest loses of weight associated with dehydration. However, it's impossible to say how much better any given athlete would perform without as much water loss. And, it can also be shown that even mild dehydration can impair muscle function. So the issue is not so simple if one wants to give general recommendation for all athletes.

What is simple is the concept of self-health management. It's quite possible that those who develop water intoxication and hyponatremia may have reduced levels of health to start with, making them most vulnerable to water intoxication and EAH. In my clinical research, going back to the late 1970s, I found many athletes who had sodium regulation problems (usually the result of hormonal imbalance). From his data, Dr. Noakes says about 10 percent of athletes may be at risk for hyponatremia due to predisposition—add to that the overconsumption of water or sports drinks and serious consequences can follow.

Athletes should take control rather than let the sports drink market set the pace of fluid recommendations. Athletes should learn the optimal way to hydrate during a long race—drinking about the same amount of water that's lost—and avoid using sports drinks as everyday beverages. Along with avoiding overtraining, and eating a proper diet, improvements in overall health helps assure proper hormone balance to better regulate water and sodium on race day—which can also contribute to a better performance.

The sensation of thirst appears after a certain degree of dehydration, and this was always interpreted as meaning thirst is not the best indicator of fluid needs. In hindsight, this may indeed be the best indicator if mild dehydration is not an issue during competition.

Primary Causes of Water Intoxication and EAH

An athlete need not consume excessively high amounts of water to develop water intoxication—it can sometimes occur with lower volumes of water intake. That's because among the real causes of the problem are 1) hormone imbalance, which reduces the ability of the body to properly regulate water; and 2) poor sodium regulation, itself controlled by other hormones. In particular, what's referred to as the *syndrome of inappropriate secretion of the antidiuretic hormone*—SIADH—has been implicated as the main cause of EAH. This involves an important brain-body mechanism called the hypothalamic-pituitary-adrenal (HPA) axis, which produces various hormones and regulates water and sodium.

While we know that serious water and sodium problems can occur in athletes during long events, it's a question of which came first—too much water, or body dysfunction that causes it. Perhaps a better question is this: *Can excess fluid intake be an aggravating factor rather than the cause of water and sodium imbalance?*

The answer to this question is "yes." While restricting fluids could save lives, it would be treating the end-result problem and not the cause. Rather than asking all athletes to reduce their water intake during endurance races, especially in hot and dry conditions where dehydration can be a factor, it would be best to also determine which individuals are susceptible to the problems of water and sodium imbalances, and correct them. While preventing ill health and death is obviously of upmost importance, the cause of the problem must still be addressed. And, whether dehydration or EAH, the responsibility of prevention lies with each athlete.

With 25 percent of Ironman finishers showing abnormally low sodium, and my observations that many more endurance athletes show some signs and symptoms of overtraining—which can adversely affect the HPA axis—the number of individuals vulnerable to this problem may be quite high.

From a health and performance standpoint, the body has a great capacity to adapt to the possibility of higher or lesser amounts of water loss in the short term, such as during a race—a reason some athletes appear to function well despite significant (less than 3 percent) water losses. This adaptation occurs because of hormones produced in the brain and body that not only regulate water, but sodium in the blood. And, consuming reasonable amounts of fluid in a healthy body should maintain some degree of water and sodium balance. But this occurs in a healthy body.

The Recipe for Disaster

Here are some key factors associated with overhydration and hyponatremia:

- Hormone imbalance, in particular the inappropriate secretion of ADH, which is produced in the brain's pituitary gland and the hypothalamus, causes poor water regulation. ADH is the body's primary regulator of water balance, informing the kidney to conserve or excrete water. Other hormones are involved as well.
- In this case, too much ADH, which can rise with the stress of a race, keeps the kidney from getting rid of water resulting in too much accumulating throughout the body. This results in weight gain.
- The HPA axis also regulates sodium via adrenal gland hormones. The result can be too much sodium loss with blood levels dropping to dangerously low levels.
- Normally, if blood sodium levels drop, reserves of this electrolyte (they're especially high in bones) should help replace that which is lost, but for unknown reasons it does not occur in those with hyponatremia.
- Overdrinking of fluids before and during a race, beyond the ability of the kidneys to excrete excess fluid, further worsens the condition. At one time people relied more on common sense when it came to drinking water in a race—dry mouth, fatigue, calculating how much might be needed based on temperature, humidity, race pace, and how many more miles remain. But with the explosion of behavioral conditioning—constant advertising by companies selling fluid replacement drinks, and encouraged by race personnel—many athletes no longer rely on their brain's natural instincts.

How can the adrenal glands, or the entire HPA axis, become dysfunctional? These mechanisms, and the production of related hormones, are significantly influenced by day-to-day training, diet and nutrition, and other lifestyle factors. Excess stress in any of these areas—including overtraining and poor diet—may impair hormone balance contributing to improper regulation of water and sodium.

From the beginning of my coaching career, I paid careful attention to sodium and its role in health and sport performance. Some athletes seemed to lose too much sodium, and this problem was found to be associated with muscle dysfunction, and bone-related problems such as stress fractures and low bone density. Hormone imbalance was a common cause as indicated by measurements of the adrenal gland's main stress hormone, cortisol. The cause of this was typically overtraining. As stress hormones increase, the levels of sex hormones fall, especially testosterone. This can further cause muscle, bone, and other problems that impair health and performance.

Whenever an athlete began working with me, I would encourage him or her to not only focus on improving fitness, but health as well so that physical, chemical and mental injuries could be avoided. Many were initially found to have subtle or sometimes more obvious hormone imbalances that reflected an impaired HPA axis. These "subclinical" problems can separate a good athlete from a great one, or an average performance from a phenomenal one.

In addition to regulating water and sodium, and the stress of training and racing, the HPA axis is associated with blood sugar control, energy production and muscle function. In particular, muscle imbalance can parallel hormone imbalance, especially the HPA axis. It's commonly known that gait irregularities are associated with hyponatremia. So a recipe for injury can be found in an athlete with muscle imbalance leading to gait irregularity and finally a local injury to a muscle or joint—along the way, reductions in performance also occur.

Various clues can provide information that a given athlete may be vulnerable to hormone imbalance associated with an impaired

HPA axis. This includes a history of bone fractures, osteoporosis or other bone injury. Others include waking in the middle of the night with difficulty getting back to sleep, increased body fat despite high levels of training, and muscle imbalance (which is often associated with many types of physical injuries).

By addressing physical, chemical, and mental stress, athletes can significantly improve their overall health and fitness, with the result of better performances and lower risks of water and sodium dysregulation.

The recipe for disaster comes when an athlete has less than adequate health as reflected by hormone imbalance and poor sodium regulation; and then, if the athlete is encouraged to drink large amounts of fluids during an event, overhydration can occur along with hyponatremia.

A simple self-assessment could help determine those at high risk for water intoxication. Weighing yourself before and after a long hard training event or especially a race, can determine changes in body weight, which reflect losses or gain in water. Any abnormal changes—weight gain or loss of more than 3 percent—should be considered a red flag that requires further evaluation.

The serious problems of water intoxication and hyponatremia should also be put in perspective to other deaths that occur during endurance events. A study published in the *British Medical Journal* (2007) examined twenty-six U.S. marathons between 1975 and 2004. Over this thirty-year period, there were twenty-four sudden cardiac deaths confirmed, with twenty-one due to atherosclerosis, four from water intoxication and hyponatremia, two due to heart abnormalities, and one from heat stroke. Virtually all these deaths were preventable.

Healthy athletes who are properly trained tend to regulate their sodium and water very well, avoiding hyperhydration and hyponatremia. In an ideal world, it's best for athletes to take responsibility for their own health to ensure they lower their risk of serious illness and death, which will also help them reach their athletic potential.